THE COLOR ATLAS OF
INTESTINAL PARASITES

By

FRANCIS M. SPENCER, A.B., M.D., F.A.C.P., F.A.C.G.

*Diplomate of the American Board of Internal Medicine, and
the Subspecialty Board of Gastro-Enterology
Active Member, American Gastroenterological Association
Gastroenterologist and Member of the Department of Internal Medicine
Angelo Clinic Association
San Angelo, Texas*

and

LEE S. MONROE, M.S., M.D., F.A.C.P., F.A.C.G.

*Diplomate of the American Board of Internal Medicine, and
the Subspecialty Board of Gastro-Enterology
Active Member, American Gastroenterological Association
Senior Consultant, Division of Gastroenterology
Scripps Clinic and Research Foundation
La Jolla, California*

With a Foreword by

Ernest Carroll Faust

*Professor of Parasitology
Tulane University School of Medicine
New Orleans, Louisiana, and
University of Valle, Cali, Colombia*

THE COLOR ATLAS OF INTESTINAL PARASITES

Second Edition

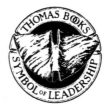

CHARLES C THOMAS • PUBLISHER

Springfield • *Illinois* • *U.S.A.*

Published and Distributed Throughout the World by

CHARLES C THOMAS • PUBLISHER

2600 South First Street, Springfield, Illinois, 62717, U.S.A.

RC
119.7
S6
1982

First Printing, 1961
Second Printing, 1966
Third Printing, 1968
Fourth Printing, 1971
Fifth Printing, 1973
Revised Sixth Printing, 1975
Seventh Printing, 1977
Second Edition, 1982

With THOMAS BOOKS *careful attention is given to all details of
manufacturing and design. It is the Publisher's desire to present books that
are satisfactory as to their physical qualities and artistic possibilities and
appropriate for their particular use.* THOMAS BOOKS *will be true to those
laws of quality that assure a good name and good will.*

Printed in the United States of America
V-C-1

Library of Congress Cataloging in Publication Data

Spencer, Francis M.
    The color atlas of intestinal parasites.

    Bibliography: p.
    Includes index.
    1. Worms, Intestinal and parasitic--Identifica-
tion. 2. Protozoa, Pathogenic--Identification.
3. Medical parasitology--Atlases. I. Monroe, Lee S.
II. Title. [DNLM: 1. Intestinal diseases, Parasitic
--Diagnosis--Atlases. 2. Parasites--Atlases. QZ 17
S845c]
RC119.7.S6   1981   616.3'4016   81-8930
ISBN 0-398-04557-7   AACR2

This book is dedicated to

DR. FLOYD THOMAS McINTIRE

Distinguished Colleague, Teacher, Friend

FOREWORD

THE authors of this Atlas have spent untold hours of dedication to the task of preparing an unusually complete and faithful series of color photomicrographs of the intestinal protozoa, helminth eggs and larvae, and objects with which these organisms are often confused. From this larger series a generous number of representative ones have been selected for reproduction in this volume. The chapters in the text have been designed with equal care, to instruct the technical laboratory worker in appropriate methods for the preparation, examination, and accurate diagnosis of human parasitic infections.

The authors are unusually well qualified by training and experience to compile this Atlas. They are clinicians who know the difficulties and pitfalls of the average laboratory diagnostician. This authoritative pictorial guide provides for the first time an opportunity for self-instruction on the part of the intelligent laboratorian who has the ambition to develop competent diagnostic ability. The Atlas faithfully reproduces essentially all of the parasite objects obtained from the intestinal tract and likely to be encountered in the clinical laboratory. The photomicrographs include a variety of forms and stages, both in the living state and those fixed, stained and mounted by standard procedures. In this respect they are more comprehesive than a complete set of permanent slide preparations.

This Atlas will be an authoritative guide for the clinical laboratory worker and the laboratory director, and it will also be helpful to the internist who is anxious to relate the laboratory findings to the symptoms exhibited by a patient. Moreover, in clinical laboratory courses in the medical school there will be a definite reference need for the Atlas.

The authors of this compendium deserve unstinted praise for their efforts, which are bound to receive wide and enthusiastic acclaim.

Ernest Carroll Faust

PREFACE

THIS color atlas represents an undertaking that is perhaps unique, in that the authors are not parasitologists, but clinicians actively engaged in the practice of internal medicine and gastroenterology. It is our clinical experience which has impressed us with the importance of parasitic infections on the one hand, and the frequency with which such intestinal infections are overlooked on the other. Comparative observations of the diagnostic parasitology performed in a large number of clinical laboratories have left no doubt that a great many cases of parasitosis remain undetected due to failure of inexperienced and inadequately trained laboratory personnel to recognize the parasites on routine stool examination.

It is equally common, and almost as dangerous, for the poorly trained technician mistakenly to report an important parasite when none is present. Such errors cause the patient to be subjected, sometimes repeatedly, to unnecessary treatment. Moreover, the physician's attention may be diverted from the true cause of the patient's illness.

Errors in accurate identification of a parasite species are common in the average clinical laboratory, and an artifact, a pseudoparasite, or a harmless commensal may be incorrectly identified as a pathogenic species. Such errors are important, for accurate species identification is often essential to successful treatment.

While serving together as medical officers in the United States Air Force, the authors were provided with an opportunity to see a great many parasitic intestinal infections and to observe the morphology and diagnostic features of a remarkable variety of parasite species. An interest in medical photography as a hobby led us to attempt to record the diagnostic morphology of the various intestinal parasites through the use of color photomicrographs, in the hope that such photomicro-

ix

graphs would be of value in teaching our own laboratory technicians to identify correctly the important parasite forms.

These photographic endeavors have been continued over a period of several years following return to civilian practice, with gradual improvement in the quality of the photomicrographs through the development of better techniques, the acquisition of finer optical equipment, and particularly through endless repetition of the photographic attempts and the discarding of countless color slides.

The equipment used in making the photomicrographs has remained exceedingly simple. A single-lens reflex camera and a microscope identical to those found in the average clinical laboratory, except for the unusually fine quality of the optical components, were employed. The use of such highly corrected optics compensated, to some degree, for the loss of detail and definition inherent in the reproduction of photomicrographs made at very high magnifications. However, the use of special techniques, lighting, or equipment that would in any way alter the appearance of the parasites from that familiar to technicians working in the ordinary clinical laboratory has been carefully avoided.

The reader should bear in mind that photomicrography at high magnificaiton is complicated by an exceedingly narrow depth of field, so that the camera records an image that is restricted to a single plane of optical focus. In several instances we have attempted to compensate for this effect, which is exaggerated in the case of the higher magnifications required for the protozoan forms, by using a series of photomicrographs of the same parasite made in successively lower focal planes. Such serial photographic studies make it possible to demonstrate the complete morphologic structure of the organism.

In May of 1958, at the World Congress of Gastroenterology in Washington, D.C., and again in June of 1958, at the Annual Meeting of the American Medical Association in San Francisco, a portion of the collection of photomicrographs was presented as a scientific exhibit intended to demonstrate their value as an aid in teaching recognition of the intestinal parasites. The recognition and enthusiastic encouragement we received from parasitologists, teachers, gastroenterologists, general practitioners, and a variety of specialists have stimulated us to make available, for teaching purposes, this more complete and comprehensive collection of our color photomicrographs.

The 256 original color photomicrographs reproduced herein demonstrate the characteristic morphology and diagnostic forms of most of the important intestinal parasites of man, *as they actually appear when viewed through the ordinary laboratory microscope.*

The protozoan parasites are all shown at a single standardized magnification (×1320), to permit immediate visual size comparisons of the various forms and species. Similarly, the diagnostic helminth eggs are all shown at an appropriately lower standard magnification (×430). A wide variety of common and confusing structures, pseudoparasites, and harmless commensals are included, each being shown at the standard magnification appropriate to its size. All magnifications have been carefully determined by measurement with a stage micrometer.

It is our sincere hope that this Color Atlas will achieve its intended purpose by serving as a practical aid in training laboratory technicians, medical students, and physicians in the recognition and accurate identification of the intestinal parasites.

FRANCIS M. SPENCER
LEE S. MONROE

ACKNOWLEDGMENTS

THE authors are deeply grateful to Dr. Ernest Carroll Faust, Professor of Parasitology at Tulane University School of Medicine, New Orleans, Louisiana, and the University of Valle, Cali, Colombia, for his generous encouragement and the invaluable assistance provided by his detailed and critical review of the entire manuscript and the complete collection of color photomicrographs.

We also offer our sincere thanks to Drs. John F. Kessel and Marietta Voge, of the School of Medicine, Univeristy of California, Los Angeles, who have given many helpful comments and suggestions. We are indebted to Dr. Kessel for the generous loan of the iron hematoxylin-stained slides from which our original color photomicrographs of *Entamoeba polecki* were made. Thanks are due Mr. Roy B. Johnson, Director of Laboratories at the Scripps Clinic and Research Foundation, for assistance in the preparation of the chapter on Laboratory Methods. We wish also to extend our thanks to Mr. L. C. Wall, of the Medical Division of the Eastman Kodak Company, for his valuable technical advice and help in checking carefully the true magnifications represented by the photomicrographs reproduced in this volume.

Perhaps the most difficult task involved in the preparation of an Atlas intended to demonstrate a complete series of the diagnostic forms of the intestinal parasites is the acquisition of material containing all of the many parasite species infecting the human intestinal tract. It is equally difficult to establish the identity of some of the unusual species included in this collection. For their invaluable assistance in these vital tasks we wish to express our sincere appreciation to Dr. Clyde Swartzwelder, Professor of Medical Parasitology of Louisiana State University School of Medicine, New Orleans; Dr. Haig Najarian, Associate Research Parasitologist for Parke, Davis & Company and

Ecologist for the World Health Organization; Dr. Mae Melvin, Parasitologist at the Communicable Disease Center Laboratory, Department of Health, Education, and Welfare, Public Health Service, Chamblee, Georgia; Dr. J. K. G. Silvey, Director and Professor of Biology and Chairman of the Division of Science at North Texas State College, Denton, Texas; and Dr. Joseph H. Miller of the Louisiana State University School of Medicine, New Orleans.

We wish to express our very special thanks and warmest gratitude to Marion C. Laufenburg, M.T., of the 3700th U.S.A.F. Hospital, Lackland Air Force Base, San Antonio, Texas, who furnished much of the material and prepared a majority of the stained smears from which our original color photomicrographs were made. Without her generous help and untiring cooperation during the past six years this volume would not have been possible.

We have drawn freely from the published literature and several textbooks of parasitology for information, and if specific credit has been omitted, we regret it. In particular we wish to acknowledge our indebtedness to the authors and publishers of *Craig & Faust's Clinical Parasitology*, 8th Ed., by E. C. Faust and P. F. Russell, Lea & Febiger, Philadephia; *Diagnostic Medical Parasitology*, by E. K. Markell and M. Voge, W. B. Saunders Company, Philadelphia; and *A Manual of Tropical Medicine*, 2nd Ed., by T. T. Mackie, G. W. Hunter III, and C. B. Worth, W. B. Saunders Company, Philadelphia.

The authors have enjoyed the most understanding cooperation and unfailing personal interest from the staff of Charles C Thomas, Publisher. For their courteous assistance and tolerant guidance we are sincerely grateful.

* * * *

In the preparation of the Revised Sixth Printing of *The Color Atlas*, the authors are indebted to I. G. Kagan, of the Center for Disease Control, Atlanta, Georgia, for a review of the section on serologic procedures; A. J. Duggan, of the Wellcome Museum of the Medical Sciences, London, England who provided additional specimens for photography; and the late S. J.

Powell, of the Amoebiasis Research Unit, Durban South Africa, for the material showing the variations in the aspirate from amebic liver abscess.

* * * *

In the preparation of the Second Edition, the authors gratefully acknowledge the cooperation of Louis S. Diamond and Carol Cunnick of the Parasitology Division of the National Institutes of Health for kindly providing axenic cultures of *Entamoeba histolytica*, which were used in the demonstration of hematophageous trophozoites. Appreciation is also expressed to the Parasite Study Group of the San Diego Zoo Hospital and particularly to Drs. G. E. Cosgrove, Andrew C. Olson, Jr., and Max Hauser for their help in preparing this most recent manuscript.

CONTENTS

THE COLOR ATLAS OF
INTESTINAL PARASITES

"CAUTIONS IN VIEWING OBJECTS"

Beware of determining and declaring your Opinion suddenly on any Object; for Imagination often gets the Start of Judgment, and makes People believe they see Things, which better Observations will convince them could not possibly be seen: therefore assert nothing till after repeated Experiments and Examinations in all Lights, and in all Positions.

When you employ the Microscope, shake off all Prejudice, nor harbour any favourite Opinions; for, if you do, it is not unlikely Fancy will betray you into Error, and make you think you see what you wish to see.

Remember, that Truth alone is the Matter you are in Search after; and if you have been mistaken, let no Vanity seduce you to persist in your Mistake.

Pass no Judgment upon Things over-extended by Force, or contracted by Dryness, or in any Manner out of their natural State, without making suitable Allowances.

—Henry Baker

Of Microscopes, and the Discoveries Made Thereby
Vol. I, Chapter XV
Read before the *Royal Society*, October 28, 1742

Chapter 1

INTRODUCTION

INFECTIONS with intestinal parasites are a medical and public health problem of growing clinical importance. Many factors have contributed to an increase in the variety as well as the incidence of parasitic infections in this country during the past three decades. Prominent among these were the Second World War, the Korean conflict, and the Vietnam War, which resulted in our military personnel being stationed in areas all around the globe where a remarkable variety of both familiar and unfamiliar intestinal parasitic diseases are endemic or hyperendemic. Environmental circumstances were such that many contracted intestinal parasites, which were at times only troublesome and at other times extremely serious.

The distribution of our armed forces continues to be worldwide, and not infrequently military personnel are accompanied by their families to remote areas where parasites abound and primitive methods of sanitation and hygiene exist. Large numbers of civilians, employed by private industry or serving with some agency of the government, also live and work in areas where they are exposed to these infections formerly regarded as exotic and unimportant to physicians practicing in this country.

Astounding increases in the speed and ease of travel have helped to stimulate an unprecedented growth in the popularity of vacation trips to foreign lands, and inevitably some travelers return home with parasites acquired while abroad. Increasing immigration, especially from Puerto Rico and neighboring areas, has contributed to the fact that we are now faced with the problem of recognizing and treating parasite infections that were previously considered rare and insignificant curiosities. For example, infection with *Schistosoma mansoni* is now one of the most prevalent parasitic diseases in New York City!

3

The true incidence of infections with the common helminths and protozoa is undoubtedly much higher than is generally suspected. This is particularly true in the case of *Entamoeba histolytica,* which is the most important of the protozoan parasites and is capable of causing serious and even fatal disease. The unsuspected high incidence of chronic amebiasis and the difficulty of diagnosis have been emphasized by many authors, although some maintain that it has been exaggerated and overemphasized. While it may be true that some statistics have greatly overestimated the incidence of chronic amebiasis, our own clinical experience has convinced us that the presence of *Entamoeba histolytica* in the stools is frequently not detected by the routine examinations performed in many clinical laboratories.

Some idea of the enormity of the parasite problem may be gained from the work of Stoll, who in 1947 carefully calculated world human helminth infections at 355 million for *Trichuris trichiura,* 35 million for *Strongyloides stercoralis,* 644 million for *Ascaris lumbricoides,* 208 million for *Enterobius vermicularis,* and 456 million for hookworm.

Yet it is the exception rather than the rule for the physician to obtain accurate and careful diagnostic work in parasitology from his clinical laboratory. Partly because of this, his index of suspicion for intestinal parasitic diseases has tended to be low. The presence of intestinal parasites remains undetected and unsuspected in a great many cases because of failure of an inexperienced or inadequately trained laboratory technician to recognize and identify them on routine stool examination. In many other instances the physician is misled by the technician reporting an important parasite when none is present. After experiencing a few such embarrassing diagnostic errors the physician may be inclined to disregard all reports of stool examinations from that laboratory; he may even discontinue altogether the practice of requesting such examinations.

The reasons for these diagnostic laboratory errors are many, not the least of which is that the technician often lacks actual experience in seeing the various intestinal parasites through his microscope. The chronic unavailability of adequate material for teaching and study makes it exceedingly difficult for technicians in many areas to gain the practical experience so vital to the development of proficiency in diagnostic parasitology. As a result, it is common for the technician to turn to the illustrations provided in the available textbooks as a means of identifying the structures seen through the microscope.

A majority of these illustrations are composite or diagrammatic drawings intended to show the diagnostic features of the parasite. Unfortunately, the medical artist may provide only a line drawing which bears little resemblance to the parasite as seen through the microscope; or he may record details that are quite invisible to the technician using standard laboratory equipment and techniques. While such drawings are very useful adjunct to teaching recognition of the intestinal parasites, they have proven to be totally inadequate and frequently misleading when the laboratorian, lacking practical experience, attempts to utilize them for making identifications.

The relatively few photomicrographs published in textbooks on parasitology or laboratory diagnosis tend to vary greatly in quality, and most are handicapped by reproduction in black and white rather than natural colors. They usually have been obtained from several different sources and are apt to represent many different magnifications, so that the technican is confused by the lack of any standard for size comparison.

The purpose of this Atlas is to provide an entirely original and virtually complete collection of color photomicrographs demonstrating the various species and stages of the intestinal parasites found in the stool of the patient, which we believe may help to solve this difficult diagnostic and teaching problem. The photomicrographs are faithfully reproduced in full-color engravings which show the parasites exactly as they appear when viewed through the laboratory microscope. Each species is shown at an appropriate standardized magnification, permitting immediate visual size comparison with similar species and with other familiar forms and structures, thus obviating the need for memorizing meaningless "average diameters" in microns. A large number of photomicrographs have been included in order to demonstrate as completely as possible the many variations in size, structure, and morphologic detail to which some species are subject.

In nearly every instance the diagnostic forms of the parasite are depicted as they appear in the fresh, unstained state, as well as when stained by several techniques and methods in common use. In most cases the photomicrographs will make it possible for the technician to identify accurately the various parasites he may encounter in his laboratory by visual comparisons alone, provided that he has properly prepared and stained the material for study.

It is necessary for the examiner to be entirely familiar with the nonpathogenic species of intestinal parasites in order to distinguish them from those which cause disease; it is equally important that he not be misled by any of the multitude of confusing objects that may be seen in virtually every fecal specimen. We have, therefore, included in the series of color photomicrographs a large number that demonstrate protozoan species that are harmless commensals, as well as a wide variety of pseudoparasites and confusing structures commonly encountered in routine examinations of the feces.

We would like to emphasize here the vital importance of each laboratory's establishing a planned diagnostic routine for the detection of the intestinal parasites, which includes the regular use of a permanent staining method. For example, the dysenteric form of amebiasis accompanied by the presence in the stools of actively motile trophozoites containing ingested erythrocytes is now known to represent only a small percentage of persons infected with *Entamoeba histolytica*. If one were to rely exclusively upon recognition of such forms, he would overlook the great majority of cases of infection with this most important parasite. Accurate and positive species identification of the protozoan parasites of the intestinal tract is dependent upon careful study of the cytological detail and nuclear structure, which are revealed only by permanent stains such as the iron hematoxylin stain or the Gomori-Wheatley trichrome stain.

The trichrome stain gives good results while requiring less experience and technical ability than does the iron hematoxylin stain. However, the difficulties of the iron hematoxylin stain have generally been much exaggerated, and the shortened and simplified technique described in Chapter 2 can easily be performed routinely in any clinical laboratory without undue expenditure of either time or effort. It provides sharper and more clearly defined demonstration of nuclear structure and cytological detail than does the trichrome stain, although either stain will produce slides that are entirely adequate for accurate diagnostic work.

The Color Atlas is intended to be a completely practical diagnostic manual for use in the clinical laboratory by the practicing medical technician, and in the classroom and training laboratory by teachers, student technicians, and medical students. The practicing physician will also find it useful, for he should be sufficiently familiar with the diagnostic features of the intestinal parasites to check the accuracy and validity of the reports coming from his laboratory.

This volume is not in any sense a textbook of parasitology, and we have made no attempt to include detailed descriptions of the adult forms, life cycles, epidemiology, pathogenesis, or treatment. However, brief comment is included regarding the distribution and pathogenicity of each species, and in some instances mention is made of predominant symptoms and pathology. Neither illustrations nor descriptions of animal parasites of man other than those which inhabit the gastrointestinal tract are included. All these subjects are beyond the scope of this book, and for these details the reader is referred to the excellent and comprehensive textbooks on clinical parasitology by Faust and Russell; Markell and Voge; Belding; Mackie, Hunter and Worth; and others.

Although we have emphasized here the failures and shortcomings of the technicians doing diagnostic parasitology in the average clinical laboratory, we would like to point out that the picture is not always so dark. The diagnostic laboratories in many hospitals, universities, and medical centers regularly provide reliable and accurate identification of the intestinal parasites, as well as superior training in diagnostic parasitology. Supported by local, state, and federal agencies there are, over the country, a great many laboratories that furnish valuable consulting services in parasitological diagnosis and at the same time train large numbers of laboratory technologists in the proper techniques of diagnostic parasitology. Moreover, it is not surprising that some of the most experienced and capable technicians in the field are serving in the laboratories of military hospitals. Because it was our good fortune to observe the exceptionally accurate and reliable work of such a technician, our interest in diagnostic parasitology was aroused, and we were stimulated to undertake the laborious collection of material and the photographic recording of species with which we have been occupied for more than a decade.

Chapter 2

LABORATORY METHODS

TECHNIQUES OF EXAMINATION FOR THE INTESTINAL PARASITES

I T is not our purpose to present in encyclopedic form all the wide variety of laboratory procedures for the detection of intestinal parasitism. There are, however, certain standardized methods that in our hands have proved satisfactory for the collection and preparation of specimens. These techniques have in common simplicity and practicality. The student, technician, and physician are urged to become thoroughly acquainted with this or a similarly reproducible methodology before exploring more laborious or exotic paths.

In particular, one should be exacting in his criteria for morphologic identification. The use of a permanent staining method for the demonstration of the protozoan forms is indispensable. Too often the inexperienced technician will make a "positive" diagnosis of a protozoan on the basis of a wet mount and thereby fall into the trap carefully baited by nature with blastocysts, phagocytes, yeasts, and other confusing pseudoparasites and artifacts.

Collection of Specimens

The collection of adequate specimens is one of the most important steps in the laboratory diagnosis of parasitosis and one which requires evaluation by the attending physician. Every clinician should have a routine for detection of the intestinal parasites and should modify this according to the demands of the situation. For example, it is important to realize that the patient with diarrhea or dysentery is more apt to pass trophozoites than the cysts of ameba. The physician should, therefore, make certain that fresh, warm stools are available for demonstration of the motile forms. On the other hand, when

9

the patient is passing formed stools, the laboratory should be alerted to search for cysts and to utilize concentration techniques.

The number of stools submitted for examination likewise depends on the index of clinical suspicion. Whereas most infections with helminths will be detected by one or two satisfactorily concentrated solid stool specimens, the discovery of a protozoon may be much more difficult, requiring repeated studies. Sawitz and Faust (1942) have stated that a single stool specimen examined by all methods will uncover less than half of *Entamoeba histolytica* infections, and that six or more examinations are necessary if 90 percent of infections are to be discovered. Alicna and Fadell (1959) recommend the study of at least three fecal specimens obtained by purgation.

The techniques of specimen collection should be varied to meet a given situation. A patient who has resided in an area where *Schistosoma mansoni* is endemic should have examination of biopsy specimens from the rectal mucosa as the procedure of choice. In the evaluation of pruritis ani, use of the Graham Scotch cellophane tape technique for the detection of *Enterobius vermicularis* is indicated. Unusal situations will require examination of aspirated material or duodenal drainage (for *Strongyloides stercoralis* or *Giardia lamblia*).

The following routine for the collection of specimens has proved useful in our hands. The number of specimens collected will depend, as indicated above, on the index of clinical suspicion and the demands of the case at hand.

1. Solid feces from a casual stool should be obtained. It is most convenient to collect this directly in a clean, waxed, cylindrical cardboard container. This receptacle should be free from soap or disinfectants. The stool specimen should be examined as soon as possible or preserved with PVA (see below). If necessary, this material may be stored under refrigeration for several days without degeneration of the cystic protozoan forms or helminth eggs. Motile trophozoites, however, will be destroyed by cold. The administration of barium, bismuth, magnesia, or oil to a patient may render the specimen unsatisfactory for examination.

2. Following the administration of a saline cathartic (such as

sodium sulfate, 15 grams, or buffered phospho-soda), at least three liquid stools are to be collected as described above and immediately sent to the laboratory for examination. The specimen should be examined while still warm. If any delay is apt to occur, a portion of each specimen should be mixed with the PVA fixative (see below). Purgation undoubtedly increases the number of positive findings but may be followed by a period of several days during which protozoa or helminth eggs are difficult to detect.

3. Proctosigmoidoscopy with examination of mucus or exudate scraped or aspirated from suspicious lesions is a valuable diagnostic adjunct. If the patient has recently had a bowel movement, it is frequently preferable to perform the examination without preliminary enemas. If necessary, an enema of tepid isotonic saline will probably least disturb the motility and form of trophozoites. Material attained with cotton swabs from rectal mucosa is, as a rule, not satisfactory, as protozoan trophozoites become lodged within the interstices of cotton and cannot be easily transferred to a slide. Material obtained is immediately placed on a *warm* slide, where it is diluted with *warm* isotonic saline preparatory to microscopic examination. Prior to microscopy, an electric heating pad turned to a low setting makes an ideal temporary storage area.

When schistosomiasis is suspected, superficial biopsies taken from several of the rectal valves are most apt to reveal the presence of eggs. Not infrequently eggs will be recovered from rectal mucosa that appears perfectly normal to gross inspection. The small bits of mucosa are floated in saline, compressed under a coverslip, and examined under the low power of the microscope.

4. The Graham Scotch cellophane tape technique is used for the detection of *Enterobius vermicularis* and is indicated for the investigation of pruritus ani, the finding of perianal excoriations, or a suspicion that the patient is infected. The cellophane tape is applied in the morning, sticky side down to the uncleansed perianal area. The adhesive side is then applied to a slide, preferably running a few drops of toluene between the tape and the slide to remove air bubbles, and examined under low power. The eggs of *Enterobius vermicularis* also may be

demonstrated with surprising regularity if the outside of a solid stool is scraped with an applicator and the material examined in a wet mount or after concentration.

5. On rare occasions other material is examined, such as duodenal aspirate, sputum, or fresh material from ulcers or abscesses. This should be studied as soon as possible to prevent degeneration of motile forms.

PREPARATION OF SPECIMENS

The Polyvinyl Alcohol (PVA) Fixative Technique

The PVA fixative technique facilitates preservation of the cysts and motile forms of the intestinal protozoa. This is of great help to the busy practitioner who does not have a reliable laboratory equipped for parasitologic diagnosis at his immediate disposal. A quantity of a stool specimen is introduced and mixed with three times or more the quantity of PVA fixative. A few drops of this mixture can then be removed at any time, perhaps months later, for the preparation of diagnostic smear. Such a slide should be allowed to dry thoroughly (preferably overnight at 37° C) before staining.

PVA fixative can also be mixed directly with a stool specimen on a slide. The 1:3 ratio of stool to fixative is maintained, and a thin smear is made. The PVA smears may be stained by any of the usual staining procedures. However, prior to routine staining, dried films are first placed in 70% ethyl alcohol containing iodine for 10 to 20 minutes in order to remove mercuric chloride crystals.

Preparation of PVA Fixative: Reagents
(1) Glacial acetic acid   5.00 ml
     Glycerol   1.50 ml
     Schaudinn's solution   93.50 ml
     (2 parts saturated aqueous solution of mercuric chloride and 1 part 95% ethyl alcohol — see under Schaudinn's solution).
(2) Polyvinyl alcohol (PVA) powder 5 grams. The modified Schaudinn's solution (1) is heated to 75° C and the PVA added while stirring.

Procedure

A quantity of the specimen is introduced into a receptacle containing PVA fixative. The 1:3 ratio of stool to fixative is retained as above. Stools can thus be preserved for months prior to staining.

Merthiolate-Iodine-Formaldehyde (MIF)
Stain and Fixative

(Sapero and Lawless)

The MIF stain and fixative is an additional simple technique by which stool preservation and staining can be accomplished simultaneously. The stock solution consists of the following:

Water	250 ml
Tincture Merthiolate No. 99	200
(Lilly) 1:1000	
Formaldehyde USP	25 ml
Glycerol	5 ml

This stock solution is stored in a brown glass bottle. Immediately prior to use, 2.35 ml of stock solution is mixed with 0.15 ml of fresh Lugol's solution (less than 1 week old), and the entire amount is mixed with approximately .25 gram of feces for bulk preservation in a well-stoppered bottle. Small amounts may then be removed at any time for examination without additional staining or fixation. Although the pink background color may be confusing when first used, this preparation gives good preservation of morphology of protozoan cysts and trophozoites.

Examination of Wet Mounts

The direct smear examination is the easiest and therefore the most frequently utilized method of examination. The technique of preparation varies slightly with the specimen. Solid feces should be sampled from several locations. Tiny portions are removed from the inside and the surface of the stool. These are transferred to a bit of heavy wax paper and therein thoroughly mixed with isotonic saline so as to give a thin suspension. Utilizing a crease in the paper, one or two drops of this mixture are poured onto a microscope slide and a coverslip placed on top. It is very important that the suspension be the proper thickness and consistency. The usual error is for the suspension to be too thick so that crowding and overlying of material prevents identification of the individual organisms. The suspension should be so thin that when the coverglass is laid upon it, it spreads smoothly and evenly across the slide. The coverglass should adhere firmly to the slide by capillary action. In liquid stools, strands of mucus are picked out with small applicator sticks, placed on a slide, and mixed with one or two drops of saline prior to examination. Thick exudate or pus usually will require dilution with saline, although a duodenal drainage sample may not. Whereas some technicians prefer the unstained slide, the study of a wet iodine-stained mount will often add much to the examination. Such a simple staining procedure will bring out additional detail in the amebic nuclei and uniformly stains the glycogen vacuole of *Iodamoeba bütschlii* a deep red-brown color. The iodine stain will often make easier the identification of some of the helminth eggs. A tiny drop of D'Antoni's iodine or dilute Lugol's is added to the stool suspension and thoroughly mixed. This stained suspension is then placed under a coverslip with the precautions noted above.

The direct smear or permanently stained film should be examined in a systematic manner. The microscopist should use an instrument with the eyepieces or objectives free from dirt or grease. It is frequently helpful to have a wide field ocular (15 or 20✕), particularly when searching for the small protozoan forms. The slide should be scanned rapidly under low power to make sure the preparation is adequate — not too thick or thin. Careful and systematic observation under low power should then begin, observing some scheme that insures that the entire slide is covered. It is suggested that the technician begin in the upper left corner of the slide and work across from left to right and back again, continuing to the lower right corner. During this period of searching, the fine focusing adjustment should be turned back and forth rapidly and slightly. Amebic cysts are highly refractile in saline or iodine-stained preparations and can often be made to "twinkle" by this maneuver. When a suspicious area is located, this is inspected under high power. In the case of permanently stained slides, it may be necessary to use the high dry objective for scanning. When a suspicious area is seen, the technician switches to the oil immersion objective to carefully study the morphologic details of the parasite.

Lugol's Solution (for direct smear staining)

Potassium iodide	10 grams
Iodide crystals	5 grams
Distilled water	100 ml

D'Antoni's Iodine — Modified

Postassium iodide	1 gram
Powdered iodine crystals	1.5 grams
Distilled water	100 ml

A potassium iodide solution is made, and powdered iodine crystals are added to saturate the solution. Undissolved iodine crystals should be present. The iodine solution is stored in the dark in a brown bottle and labeled as "stock solution." Small amounts of the stock solution can be diluted and placed in the dropper bottle for laboratory use. The laboratory solution lasts approximately twenty-four hours and should then be replaced. The stock solution is good as long as iodine crystals are seen.

Concentration of Feces

A higher percentage of positive examinations, for both the helminths and the protozoa, will result if a concentration technique is added to the routine of examination. The formalin-ether method is suggested because of its simplicity and because of the fact that it is more apt to demonstrate the larger eggs.

Formalin-Ether Concentration (Method of Ritchie)

1. Mix stool with 10 volumes of tap water;

2. Strain through gauze into 15 ml centrifuge tubes;

3. Centrifuge the strained emulsions (1 minute at 2000 r.p.m.); decant supernate;

4. Wash the sediments with tap water;

5. Repeat the centrifuging and the washing;

6. Decant the supernatant fluid;

7. Add 10 ml of 7.5% formalin to the sediment;

8. Let stand for 10 to 30 minutes;

9. Add about 3 ml of ether, stopper the tubes, and shake vigorously;

10. Centrifuge at 1500 r.p.m. for about 1 minute;

11. Free the superficial debris from the tube wall with an applicator;

12. Decant the supernatant mixture;

13. Examine the sediment under a microscope;

14. Add a tiny drop of iodine solution and examine again.

It is to be noted that permanent staining techniques using the Gomori-Wheatley trichrome stain or iron hematoxylin method cannot be used following concentration.

Modified Zinc Sulfate Concentration (Flotation)

This concentration technique has the disadvantage that it does not recover the larger operculated eggs or those of the other schistosomes; however, it is superior to others in the recovery of the ova of *E. vermicularis* and *H. nana*. The concentrate produced by this method is adequate for most clinical usages and is quite clear of detritus.

Zinc Sulfate Solution

Zinc Sulfate, USP	333 grams
Distilled water (warm)	1000 ml

The specific gravity of the above solution should be adjusted to 1.18 by appropriate additions of either zinc sulfate or water.

Technique

1. Prepare a fecal suspension in a standard centrifuge tube by

thoroughly stirring 1 volume feces in 15 of water.

2. Centrifuge for 1 minute at 2500 r.p.m. and decant the supernate. Repeat this washing if the stool is extremely oily.

3. Add zinc sulfate solution until the tube is half full and break up the sediment with an applicator stick. Then fill the tube with zinc sulfate solution.

4. Centrifuge this suspension for 1 minute at 2500 r.p.m. Do not brake the centrifuge in stopping, and avoid jarring the tube.

5. Using a bacteriological loop, remove one or two loopfuls of material floating on the surface and transfer them to a clean slide.

6. Cover specimen with a coverslip and examine directly or with a tiny drop of iodine stain.

Permanent Staining Methods

Permanent stains are necessary in order to differentiate related species of the protozoa and to serve as a record to document an infection.

Modified Iron Hematoxylin Stain

The iron hematoxylin is by far the most widely used and accepted technique. This permanent staining method gives maximum detail and allows a more reliable identification than any other method. This modified procedure does not require decolorization and is only slightly more time consuming than the Gemori-Wheatley trichrome stain.

1. Make a smear of normal saline emulsified feces, spreading thinly; place the slide in working Schaudinn's solution[1] before the smear dries;

2. Allow the slide to stand in the Schaudinn's solution for at least 1 hour. The slide may be left overnight if desirable;

---

[1]Schaudinn's solution: Make 200 ml of a saturated solution of mercuric chloride, by mixing 11.4 grams of mercuric chloride of 200 ml distilled water. Add 100 ml of 95% ethyl alcohol to the 200 ml of saturated mercuric chloride solution. This stock solution will keep practically indefinitely. From the *stock* solution, a *working* solution is made, which is good for two weeks. This is made by adding 3 ml of glacial acetic acid to 47 ml of the stock solution and mixing them thoroughly.

3. Transfer the slide to a 70% iodine-alcohol solution for approximately 5 minutes to remove the mercuric chloride crystals. (The iodine-alcohol solution is made by adding a few drops of 3% iodine to 70% alcohol);

4. Transfer slides to 95% alcohol for about 5 minutes;

5. Transfer slides to 70% alcohol for about 5 minutes;

6. Transfer slides to a Coplin jar and allow tap water to flow gently over the slides for approximately 10 minutes;

7. Place slides in a *working* solution of iron hematoxylin staining solution[2] for 4 to 5 minutes;

8. Transfer to a Coplin jar and allow tap water to flow for 10 minutes.

9. Change the slide to 70% alcohol for 5 minutes;

10. Transfer the slide to 95% alcohol for 5 minutes;

11. Place the slide in a 100% (absolute) alcohol for 5 minutes;

12. Transfer the slide to xylene (xylol) for 10 minutes;

13. Cover wet film with Clarite®, Permount® or Canada Balsam, then mount with a clean, dry No. 1 coverglass.

The slide should not be allowed to become dry at any time. The balsam should be applied while the slide is still wet with the xylene. If a chalky precipitate forms in the xylene when the slide is transferred from absolute alcohol, it indicates that dilution of the alcohol has occurred. Slides can then be cleared by first placing them in fresh absolute alcohol and then in fresh xylene.

The Trichrome (Gomori-Wheatley) Stain

As is true of the iron hematoxylin stain, the trichrome stain may be used for PVA preserved or fresh stool fixed with Schaudinn's. With this method, rapid staining can be accomplished

---

[2]Iron hematoxylin staining solutions:

    Solution (1) Hematoxylin 10 grams in 1000 ml of absolute alcohol.
             This is allowed to sit in the light for one week.

(2):		
Ferrous ammonium sulfate	10 grams
Ferric ammonium sulfate	10 grams
Concentrated hydrochloric acid	10 ml
Distilled water	1000 ml

    This solution will keep for approximately 6 months.
For preparation of the working solution of iron hematoxylin, mix carefully 15 ml each of solutions (1) and (2). This working solution will last for about 7 days.

for the identification of various intestinal protozoa. It demonstrates acceptably the cytoplasmic and nuclear details.

Technique

1. Place the Schaudinn's fixed smear
   in iodine-alcohol   1 minute;
2. In alcohol 70%   1 minute;
3. In alcohol 70%   1 minute;
4. In Gomori stain[1]   8 to 15 minutes;
5. In alcohol (90%) with
   1% acetic acid   10 to 15 seconds;
6. In alcohol 100 percent   rinse twice;
7. In alcohol 100 percent
   (fresh absolute)   30 seconds;
8. In xylol   1 minute;
9. In balsam (Technicron® mounting
   medium), Clarite®, or Permount®   until dry.

The slides can be stained rapidly and individually by moving them through a series of jars containing the proper reagents. By placing the slides in a single jar and adding and in turn decanting the successive solutions, the same result can be achieved. The iodine-alcohol and stain are retained, while the other solutions may be discarded. It is well to withdraw the slide from the acidulated 90% alcohol at intervals until the excess stain no longer flows from the slide. It is then rinsed twice in the first 100% alcohol and is then placed for 30 seconds in the second 100% alcohol. Care must be taken to maintain the concentration of the last alcohol solution, as a slight dilution will often cause clouding of the slides.

Microscopically, the background elements will be seen to stain predominantly red or green, while the

---

[1]Gomori stain is constituted from

Chromotrope 2R	.6 grams
Light green SF	.3 grams
Phosphotungstic acid	.7 grams
Acetic acid	1.00 ml
Distilled water	100.00 ml

the protozoa will take on a more neutral color — usually gray or pale green. Chromatoidal bodies and erythrocytes will take both the red and the green stains, appearing in strong contrast to the cytoplasm. Nuclear elements stain darkly.

Cultivation of Intestinal Protozoa

The technique for cultivation of the intestinal protozoa, while time consuming, will often increase the number of positive findings. Although a wide variety of media are available, it is advisable to become familiar with a selected few.

Modified Boeck and Drbohlav's Media

This media is quite time consuming to prepare and is particularly good for the transfer of amebae from one culture to another.

Preparation of Egg Slant Culture Tubes

1. Four fresh eggs are washed, broken into an electric blender containing 50 ml of Locke's solution (see below), and the mixture emulsified.
2. The mixture is then filtered through gauze, and slants are made in 15 × 125 ml sterile test tubes. The butt should be short and the slant measure approximately 4 to 5 cm.
3. The slants are placed in the autoclave at 15 pounds pressure for 15 minutes. Remember that sudden drops in pressure will cause bubbles to form in the solid slanted base.
4. Allow the slants to cool and overlay to a depth of 5 to 6 cm with Locke's solution.
5. Sterilize in an autoclave at 15 pounds pressure for 15 minutes. Release the pressure gradually.
6. Incubate for 25 hours at 37° C and check for sterility. Fresh medium is more satisfactory, but if necessary it can be stored for a month in the refrigerator.
7. Before inoculating the medium, add to each tube a tiny pinch of sterile rice powder (dried in a drying oven for 2 1/2

hours at 150° C).

Modified Locke's Solution (Overlay)

Sodium chloride	8.00 grams
Calcium chloride	0.20 grams
Potassium chloride	0.20 grams
Magnesium chloride	0.01 grams
Sodium phosphate	2.00 grams
Sodium bicarbonate	0.40 grams
Potassium phosphate	0.30 grams

1. Add and mix until dissolved the above chemicals, in the order listed, to 1000 ml of distilled water.
2. Boil 10 minutes. A precipitate will form.
3. Cool to room temperature and filter.
4. Pour the clear liquid supernate into suitable containers and sterilize in an autoclave 15 minutes at 15 pounds (121° C).

Cleveland and Collier's Medium

This medium is quite satisfactory for routine laboratory use and consists of a solid liver infusion slant with an overlay of saline and fresh serum (either horse, human, or rabbit).

Preparation of Agar Slants

1. Dissolve 30 grams of dehydrated liver infusion agar (Difco) and 3 grams of sodium phosphate in 100 ml of distilled water. The resulting solution contains —

Infusion of 272 grams of beef liver in 1000 ml of water	
Peptone	5.5 grams
Sodium chloride	2.7 grams
Disodium phosphate	3.0 grams
Agar	11.0 grams

2. Prepare agar slants 4 to 5 cm long without a butt.

3. Sterilize at 121°C for 20 minutes.
4. Add the overlay to cover the slant.
5. A tiny pinch of sterile rice starch is added before use.

It is advantageous, when only occasional cultures are desired, to use dehydrated base medium, which can be purchased.[1]

It is well to keep a few tubes in the incubator at all times as they must be 37° C before inoculation. Cultures should be examined at 24 and 48 hours before being reported as negative. To obtain material for microscopic examination, a 1 ml pipette is used. The end is closed with a forefinger, and the tip is lowered to the level of the slant. The slant is gently scraped with the pipette tip, and a few drops are allowed to enter. One or two drops are then placed on a clean slide and covered with a coverslip. The slide is warmed for several minutes in an incubator or other suitable warming device prior to examination.

The Serologic Diagnosis of Intestinal Parasitosis

Although for the most part coprologic studies are the mainstay of parasitic diagnosis, there are occasional situations in which stool studies are of little or no value. Within recent years serologic techniques have been developed that assist the physician in the diagnosis of certain intestinal parasitic infections. Evaluation of the results requires a knowledge of the natural history of the particular infection and the reliability of the tests being used. Several of these procedures, namely the agar gel diffusion precipitin (immunodiffusion) and latex agglutination for amebiasis, are practical for the average hospital or clinical laboratory. Serological tests can be obtained through the Parasitology Division of the Center for Disease Control, Atlanta, Georgia (Table I), by submitting specimens to the State Health Department or by contacting the Division directly.

---

[1]Bacto Entamoeba Medium, Digestive Ferments Co. of Detroit, Michigan.

Table I

Parasitic Disease	Tests Available	Diagnostic Titre
Amebiasis	CF, LA, IIF, I, IP, CCE, IHA*	≥ 1:256
Ascariasis	CF, BF, IHA, ELISA*	≥ 1:32
Clonorchiasis	CF, IHA	
Cysticercosis	IHA*	≥ 1:64
Echinococcis	CF, BF, LA, I, IP, CCE, IHA*	≥ 1:256
Fascioliasis	CF, IIF, IHA*	≥ 1:128
Giardiasis	IIF (experimental)	≥ 1:16
Schistosomiasis	CF, BF, IHA, P, IIF*	≥ 1:16
Strongyloidiasis	IHA*	≥ 1:64
Toxocariasis	BF, IHA, ELISA,	≥ 1:32

Tests available: Complement fixation (CF); Bentonite flocculation (BF); Indirect hemagglutination (IHA); Latex agglutination (LA); Indirect immunofluorescence (IIF); Immunodiffusion (I); Immunoelectrophoresis (IP); Countercurrent electrophoresis (CCE); Enzyme-linked immunoassay (ELISA). Diagnostic titre of tests indicated *. From data supplied by Parasitology Division, Center for Disease Control, Atlanta, Georgia.

Amebiasis

Serologic techniques for the detection of amebic infection have been available for many years. The tests first developed fell into disuse because of the nonspecificity of the amebic antigen. With the development of axenic or bacteria-free antigen by Diamond, antigen of high specificity and reliability has been developed. Preparation of antigens and the current methods for serologic study and amebiasis are well outlined by Kagan and Norman.

AGAR GEL DIFFUSION. Of the methods currently available, the agar gel diffusion precipitin test is one of the most reliable and simple to perform, and axenic antigens are commercially available.* The test is usually performed on an agar gel plate or

*Hyland Laboratories, Costa Mesa, California.
ICN Medical Diagnostic Products Division, Portland, Oregon.

agar-coated microscope slide, which contains the standard series of wells for the Ouchterlony technique. Undiluted antigen is placed in the center well, and unknown serum and positive and negative controls are placed at the outer wells. After forty-eight hours the slide is read for the formation of precipitin bands, and the slide is washed and stained with amidoblack to develop contrast and facilitate interpretation. With a positive test the precipitin line formed between the center antigen-containing well and the unknown should blend with the positive control to form the line of identification.

Although uncommonly a patient is found who does not form antibodies in response to amebic invasion, in the presence of amebic hepatic abscess (extraintestinal amebiasis) the agar gel diffusion test is positive in more than 98 percent of cases. Although the degree of positivity with symptomatic intestinal amebiasis is variable, probably depending upon the variable criteria for such a diagnosis, the reports vary from 70 to 90 percent. In the absence of tissue invasion (commensal state), the agar gel diffusion will be positive in less than 50 percent. A positive serologic test does not necessarily indicate current infection but may reflect ancient clinically unimportant disease. A negative test, however, is of definite value in excluding amebiasis as a diagnosis when extraintestinal involvement is under consideration. In the United States, where the background of ancient infection is quite low, a positive test is practically always associated with the presence of invasive amebiasis.

LATEX AGGLUTINATION. The latex agglutination test can be performed with simple materials and has the advantage of speed: a result can be obtained in approximately 35 minutes. The test is performed with antigen-coated latex particles and positive, negative, and unknown sera. Before testing, the sera is inactivated by heat (30 minutes at 56° C), and one drop of each serum sample is added to one drop of the latex antigen in suspension and mixed with a glass rod. In addition, as a nonspecific control, uncoated latex is mixed with unknown serum and handled similarly. In a negative test, latex particles remain uniformly distributed throughout the droplet. A positive test shows definite macroscopic clumping of the latex particles with intervening clear areas. If the known sera agglutinates uncoated latex, the test is read as indeterminate. In general, the sensitivity of the latex agglutination is comparable to that of the agar gel diffusion. The chief limiting factor is the false-positive reactions that occur in approximately 5 percent of cases, and the bulk of these are occasioned by the presence of rheumatoid factor in the serum. A commercial source of the latex agglutination test is available.*

COUNTERELECTROPHORESIS. Counterelectrophoresis has recently been developed as a serologic test and apparently has the same degree of sensitivity as the agar gel diffusion, the indirect hemagglutination, and latex agglutination. False-positive reactions are negligible. Equipment is costly; however, the results can be obtained in approximately one hour. The antigen and a commercial source for the equipment are available.†

INDIRECT HEMAGGLUTINATION. The indirect hemagglutination test is reliable and positive in over 95 percent of cases with amebic hepatic abscess and 85 percent of those with symptomatic intestinal amebiasis. The methodology is, however, laborious and has the disadvantage of requiring a supply of fresh sheep red cells. An IHA titer of 1:128 or greater is considered significant. As a rule, a negative test is found in the commensal state. The test requires clinical interpretation, as old healed infections will leave the patient with a positive serology for months to years. It is seldom that the indirect hemagglutination test is done by laboratories other than those specializing in the detection of parasitic diseases.

THE COMPLEMENT FIXATION. The technique for the performance of the complement fixation is laborious, and in most laboratories, it has been abandoned for the agar gel precipitin, which gives essentially the same results. The complement fixation test is somewhat less reactive than the indirect hemagglutination and becomes negative, as a rule, within a year or two after an acute infection. In the presence of noninvasive amebiasis (commensal state), the test is usually negative.

THE FLUORESCENT ANTIBODY TECHNIQUE. This technique is finding increasing favor as a specific diagnostic method. Essentially, the test depends upon the finding of serum antibodies

---

*Sera Ameba, Miles Laboratories, Elkhart, Indiana.
†Hyland Laboratories, Costa Mesa, California

which attach to the surface of the trophozoites of *Entamoeba histolytica*. The test requires a supply of *E. histolytica* trophozoites, which are dried on a slide. Fluoresceinated antihuman globulin is used to demonstrate the binding of antibody to the trophozoite. The technique requires ultraviolet microscopy and has approximately the same sensitivity as indirect hemagglutination and the agar gel diffusion. The indirect fluorescent antibody technique has also proved useful in demonstrating the presence of *Entamoeba histolytica* within tissues.

ENZYME-LINKED IMMUNOSORBENT ASSAY. This technique is under investigation for the recognition of antibody in serum, stool, and abscess fluid. The test utilizes an antiglobulin-peroxidase conjugate, which adheres to antibody bound to antigen, which in turn is bound to polystyrene. After washing, the residual peroxidase linked to this antigen-antibody-antiglobulin system oxidizes a suitable substrate (usually 2-amino-2-hydroxysalicylic acid) to produce a color change. The method appears sensitive, but bacterial and tissue peroxidases produce false-positive results. Clinical data are as yet meager.

Giardiasis

INDIRECT IMMUNOFLUORESCENCE. Recently an immunofluorescence test has been developed to detect antibodies to *Giardia lamblia*. Trophozoite-coated slides provide the antigen, and the antigen-antibody binding is identified with fluoresceinated antihuman globulin. In preliminary studies, antibodies have been identified in more than 90 percent of known symptomatic cases, and titers of greater than 1:16 are believed significant.

Nematodes

Coprology remains the mainstay for the diagnosis of the intestinal roundworms. A number of serologic studies are, however, currently under evaluation as an aid to the diagnosis of nematode infection (Table I). Such procedures are often hampered by the cross reactivity of the available antigens. Of value but beyond the scope of this book are the serologic tests for the diagnosis of invasion by the tissue-inhabiting roundworms, the larve of *Trichinella spiralis*, and visceral larva migrans (*Toxocara canis* and *T. cati*). The latter techniques are well outlined by Kagan and Norman.

Ascariasis

Serology is unreliable in the diagnosis of ascariasis, and proven cases may be negative. Owing to a high degree of cross reactivity, antigen extracts of both *Ascaris lumbricoides* and *Toxocara canis* are employed in the performance of the bentonite flocculation and precipitin tests (Kagan and Norman). A specific diagnosis can occasionally be reported on the basis of differential titers or by absorption techniques.

Cestodes

It is only with tissue invasion by cestode larva that serologic tests become of value, and in the majority of *Taenia saginata* and *T. solium* intestinal infections, patients are seronegative.

Cysticercosis

An important exception to the rule occurs when man becomes the intermediate host to *T. saginata* and *T. solium*. Although cases are scarce, the hemagglutination and gel diffusion precipitin tests may give positive results. A complement fixation test is available but is the least reliable, lacking sensitivity and specificity. In a titer of greater than 1:128, the hemagglutination test yields approximately 75 percent positive results in proven cases, whereas the gel diffusion precipitin is of lesser sensitivity. Patients with intestinal infections with *T. saginata* and *T. solium* but without cystocercosis may give positive serology in about 15 percent. Cross reactions occur with echinococcus and coenurus infections (Kagan and Norman).

Echinococcus

The serologic diagnosis of echinococcus disease is usually made by the indirect hemagglutination and bentonite flocculation tests. The indirect hemagglutination is considered to be of greater sensitivity than the bentonite flocculation, and titers of 1:128 and 1:5, respectively, are deemed positive. In patients with a proven diagnosis, approximately 85 percent with hepatic and 40 percent with pulmonary cysts have a significant titer. Approximately 10 percent of patients ill with other diseases will give a positive test (Kagan and Norman).

The skin test, the Casoni test, is approximately as sensitive as the indirect hemagglutination test but is less specific. Following the intracutaneous injection of 0.05 of a standardized skin test antigen, the production in 20 minutes of a wheal area with pseudopodia measuring 1.2 mm² or more is considered positive.

Trematodes

A complement fixation test is available* for the diagnosis of clonorchiasis and fascioliasis; however, data regarding the reliability are scarce. As *F. hepatica* finds man a rather resistant host, stool studies may be negative. In the appropriate classical setting, serology should prove an important diagnostic aid.

Schitosomiasis

A complement fixation and indirect immunofluorescent test are available.* Both procedures are positive in approximately 90 percent of cases with schistosomiasis and 5 percent with trichinosis. Specificity is very high except for trichinosis. Stool or biopsy studies are preferred for diagnosis and species determination.

---

*Center for Disease Control, Atlanta, Georgia.

Chapter 3

THE INTESTINAL PROTOZOA

THE AMEBAE

Entamoeba histolytica

THE most important of the protozoa infecting the digestive tract of man is *E. histolytica*. The pathogenicity of this ameba is unquestioned, and its ability to invade and destroy tissue is well established. While a chronic form of amebiasis, frequently unaccompanied by significant clinical symptoms, is more common in this country than the dysenteric form of the disease, it is essential to keep in mind that this parasite is always capable of producing serious and even fatal disease. The organisms localize in the colon, chiefly the cecum. Following invasion, metastatic lesions may appear in the liver, lung, and occasionally the brain, rarely the skin.

A long-standing controversy centers about the significance of "small" and "large" races of *E. histolytica*. Investigators in recent years emphasize that careful measurements reveal two separate strains of *E. histolytica*, which are morphologically similar but differ greatly in disease-producing potential. The nonpathogenic small race *E. histolytica*, otherwise known as *Entamoeba hartmanni*, has cysts which are regularly less than 10 microns in diameter and trophozoites which are nonhematophageous. In addition, to add further confusion, certain ameba (Laredo strain), morphologically indistinguishable from *E. histolytica*, can be separated by their ability to grow at room temperature and in hypotonic media. Laredo strain has not been incriminated in any disease process. We do not wish to participate in this dispute and observe that the average hospital laboratory is not capable of reliably making the differentiation. We must emphasize that it is never safe to assume that *E. histolytica* is harmless, regardless of the average size of cysts obtained from a given individual. In any case, the implications

29

regarding the previous environment and contacts of the host, as well as the public health aspects of the problem, cannot be ignored.

Although infections with *E. histolytica* are more common in tropical and subtropical areas, the disease is worldwide in distribution. The incidence in our own country, as well as in other areas that pride themselves on their superior methods and practice of sanitation and personal hygiene, is substantial. There is great variation in statistics reporting the incidence of amebiasis in various parts of the United States, as well as in other areas all over the globe. When one considers all the differences in diagnostic techniques, it is hardly surprising that the reported incidence in a given geographic locale may vary from less than 2 to more than 50 percent. The variation in the methods of collection and examination, the number and type of persons included and specimens examined in a given series, and the environmental circumstances of the population sampled all produce variables peculiar to such statistical reports. It is probable that the relatively high incidence reported by expert parasitologists in numerous surveys is a much more accurate reflection of the true frequency of amebiasis than are the impressions gained by physicians in private practice from the small number of cases discovered in their own clinical laboratories.

Sawitz and Faust (1942) have pointed out that less than half the cases of *E. histolytica* infection will be discovered if a single stool is examined, even though saline and iodine mounts, zinc sulfate concentration, and the iron hematoxylin stain are employed in the examination. If only saline and iodine mounts are examined, less than 20 percent will be found! But if all techniques, including the iron hematoxylin stain, are utilized, approximately 80 percent of the infections will be uncovered by the examination of three stools, and more than 90 percent if six stool specimens are examined!

We cannot emphasize too strongly the importance of the regular and routine utilization of a permanent staining method as an indispensable step in the examination of feces in every clinical laboratory where diagnostic parasitology is attempted. Without such stains, the number of protozoan parasites discovered will be a small fraction of those actually present, and many pseudoparasites and harmless commensals will be mistakenly reported as important pathogens. Accurate species identification must be made by careful study of the morphology and details of nuclear structure that are visible only in preparations stained by iron hematoxylin, the Gomori-Wheatley trichrome stain, or one of the other permanent stains. In a substantial number of cases, even the experienced and well-trained examiner will find it essential to rely on the permanent stains for positive confirmation of diagnostic suspicions and impressions gained from study of the saline and iodine mounts. Moreover, the stained slides provide an invaluable permanent record that can be mailed to a consulting laboratory.

Trophozoites of *Entamoeba histolytica* in freshly passed stools exhibit active motility by means of pseudopodia — long digitiform extensions of the ectoplasm into which the endoplasm flows. A pseudopod may be formed anywhere on the surface of the organism and may be retracted as rapidly when environmental factors dictate a change in the direction of movement or a temporary period of inactivity. Movement may appear to be directional and purposeful, but at other times it appears to be erratic. It may be continuous or intermittent, and the speed of locomotion varies with the temperature and other conditions affecting the environment of the ameba; however, movement is never long continued in a straight line.

The motility exhibited by *E. histolytica* trophozoites is best described as *flowing*. It is unfortunate that at times words such as "trip hammer" have been used to describe the action of its pseudopodia, for such terms are extremely misleading and have caused a great deal of confusion among students and inexperienced examiners.

In fresh, unstained preparations, the clear hyaline ectoplasm forming the outer layer of the body of the ameba is easily distinguished from the more centrally located and more granular endoplasm. It is also possible at times to distinguish the ectoplasm from the finely granular endoplasm in preparations well stained with iron hematoxylin. When red blood cells are recognized within the cytoplasm, they are a reliable guide to accurate identification of the trophozoite as *E. histolytica* and indicate that the protozoan has invasive qualities. In the unstained tropozoite, the erythrocytes appear as pale, refractile, greenish or colorless discoid bodies. In slides stained with iron hematoxylin, ingested red cells are stained a deep blue-black color and are seen to vary somewhat in size, shape, and intensity of staining, according to the degree to which they have been affected by the digestive process. When the trichrome stain is used, freshly ingested erythrocytes appear bright pink or red in color but quickly darken and fade as digestion proceeds. Bacteria are not normally ingested by the trophozoites of this species.

The nucleus is invisible or is seen with great difficulty in unstained trophozoites of *E. histolytica*. Details of nuclear structure are clearly seen only in slides stained with iron hematoxylin or a similar permanent stain. The single, spherical nucleus possesses a compact and punctiform karyosome, which is typically central in position. The inner surface of the distinct but delicate nuclear membrane is lined by an accumulation of chromatin granules, which are classically minute and evenly distributed. However, these chromatin deposits may form larger aggregates of granules appearing as plaquelike masses, which may be evenly or irregularly distributed. It is sometimes possible to see delicate and lightly stained fibrils between the karyosome and the chromatin of the nuclear membrane.

SEE COLOR PLATES I, II, AND III FOR PHOTOMICROGRAPHS DEMONSTRATING THE TROPHOZOITES OF *Entamoeba histolytica.*

Cysts of *E. histolytica* appear as hylaine, spherical bodies in unstained fresh smears. The very refractile cyst wall, or membrane, helps to distinguish amebic cysts from many of the pseudoparasites and artifacts with which they might be confused. The nuclei of unstained cysts may not be visible, but at times they can be recognized as a delicate ring of granules surrounding a punctate karysome in the center of the nucleus. The cytoplasm is either slightly refractive and colorless or a pale greenish color. By their smooth and refractive surfaces, which may stand out quite clearly, chromatoidal bodies may sometimes be recognized in the cytoplasm.

When stained with iodine, the cysts are bright greenish

yellow or yellow-brown in color, and the cytoplasm loses its lustrousness and appears to be finely granular. Nuclei are quite clearly seen, appearing as a dark ring of delicately beaded, refractive granules. The nuclear karyosome is punctate, and while it is more often centrally disposed, it is not infrequently eccentrically located within the nucleus. One to four nuclei may be present. Chromatoidal bodies stain poorly with iodine but can usually be distinguished, if present, from the more granular and less refractive cytoplasm. Glycogen present in the vaculoes will be stained a deep reddish brown.

In preparations stained with iron hematoxylin or the trichrome stain, the cyst wall remains unstained, so that the organism appears to be surrounded by a conspicuous clear zone. This clear zone is a useful landmark, helping to distinguish the protozoan cysts when scanning the stained slides. It is present in both mature and immature cysts of all amebae, as well as the flagellates, but is not seen in the trophozoites or the precysts.

Cysts of *E. histolytica* contain from one to four nuclei; very rarely are cysts of this species found to contain more than four nuclei, and for practical purposes the phenomenon may be disregarded. The peripheral chromatin ring lining the nuclear membrane is apt to be thicker and less uniform than in the trophozoites, and the nuclear karyosome is less reliably central in position. In slides stained with iron hematoxylin, all nuclear structures are a deep bluish-black color. When the trichrome stain is used, nuclear chromatin is also dark red or dark greenish blue in color, often appearing to be black, though less intensely so than in cysts stained with iron hematoxylin.

The young cysts contain a single large nucleus, which frequently exhibits abundant and coarse chromatin granules lining the nuclear membrane, and heavy, rather dispersed karyosomal chromatin. As nuclear division occurs, binucleate as well as trinucleate and mature quadrinucleate cysts are produced. The size of the nucleus progressively diminishes as the number of nuclei is increased.

It is useful to recognize the difference between a nucleus in repose and a nucleus in a state of activity. A nucleus showing evidence of karyokinetic activity is characterized by its large size, dispersal of coarse karyosomal chromatin, and by the heavy deposits of chromatin lining the nuclear membrane. The nucleus may be spherical but is more likely to be elongate, ovoid, elliptical, or even fusiform in shape. By contrast, the resting nucleus is small, nearly always spherical in shape, and possesses a delicate nuclear membrane lined by fine granules of chromatin and a tiny, compact karyosome.

By recognizing these variations in nuclear activity, it may be possible to distinguish a mature from an immature cyst. When four nuclei are present, a problem in the differential diagnosis between *E. histolytica* and *E. coli* may arise. If the cyst is small and four small, spherical nuclei of equal size are present, it is almost certainly a mature quadrinucleate cyst of *E. histolytica*. If four nuclei of unequal size are present, or if one or more of the nuclei reveals evidence of karyokinetic activity as described above, it is reasonable to assume that nuclear division is still incomplete and the cyst is immature. Upon completion of mitosis, the cyst will probably contain eight nuclei and is almost sure to be a cyst of *E. coli*. Diagram 1 depicts the nuclear morphology of the cysts and trophozoites of *E. histolytica*.

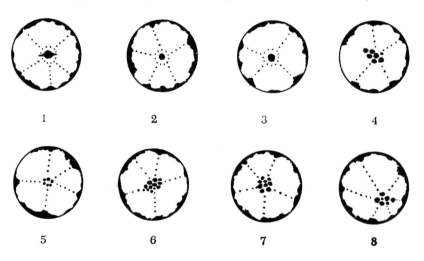

Diagram 1. Variations in nuclear morphology of *E. histolytica*: trophozoites (1 through 3) and cysts (4 through 8).

The cytoplasm of cysts of *E. histolytica* stained with iron hematoxylin is composed of very fine granules, which are, however, irregularly distributed. The result is an alveolar, spongy, and often vacuolated appearance, which is sufficiently characteristic to be of definite value in differential diagnosis.

A large glycogen vacuole may occupy most of the body of the very young cyst, appearing as a clear space in preparations stained with iron hematoxylin or the trichrome stain. Surrounding the glycogen vacuole, large numbers of small chromatoidal bodies are often arranged at the periphery of the cyst. Such immature cysts are most often uninucleate or binucleate, and regularly possess large nuclei showing evidence of karyokinetic activity. In these immature cysts there is little in the details of nuclear structure, shape, or arrangement of the chromatoidals or characteristics of the cytoplasm that is of assistance in the differential diagnosis between *E. histolytica* and *E. coli*. Even the size of the cysts is not a reliable criterion, and for accurate species identification it is usually necessary to rely upon the diagnostic features present in more mature cysts found on the same slide.

The chromatoidals present and their staining capacity tend to decrease as the cysts ripen and quite often are not found in the mature, quadrinucleate cysts. The chromatoidal bodies are classically rod shaped or elongate in this species and have blunt or rounded ends. However, the chromatoid bars may be short and thick, thin and curved, oval to nearly spherical, or extremely irregular in shape, but not with aciculate ends as in cysts of *E. coli*. The chromatoidals are stained a deep blueblack by the iron hematoxylin, whereas with the trichrome stain they appear varying shades of pale or bright pink.

The pronounced variations in the size of cysts of *E. histolytica* are well demonstrated in the color photomicrographs.

SEE COLOR PLATES IV, V, VI, AND VII FOR PHOTOMICROGRAPHS DEMONSTRATING THE CYSTS OF *Entamoeba histolytica.*

Aspirate from an amebic liver abscess has certain physical features which should be recognized. Although in many texts the material is classically reported to resemble "anchovy sauce," the description does not apply to the color of the aspirate when first removed. In an acute abscess (one with symptoms of less that 2 weeks' duration), on initial exposure to air the color is reddish or a marbled red and only with the passage of time, 30 minutes or more, does the dark brown to brown-black coloration develop. The aspirate has a custardlike consistency and if placed on gauze will not sink into the material. The material is odorless — an important differential in separating an uncomplicated amebic abscess from a bacterial or secondarily infected lesion, which, due to the presence of anaerobes, is characteristically foul-smelling. With long-standing infection, fluid gradually becomes thinner in consistency, and after more than 3 months the color may be light yellow. Inasmuch as trophozoites are encountered in the highest concentration in the last bit of material aspirated, this portion should be submitted for microscopy and culture.

SEE COLOR PLATES **XXXIII** AND **XXXIV** FOR PHOTOGRAPHS DEMONSTRATING VARIATIONS IN THE ASPIRITE FROM AMEBIC LIVER ABSCESS.

Entamoeba coli

Entamoeba coli is a nonpathogenic ameba found in a large percentage of persons examined in all parts of the world. Although this cosmopolitan parasite is a harmless commensal in the digestive tract of man, it is essential that it be distinguished from *E. histolytica,* which it closely resembles. Accurate differential diagnosis is necessary in order that appropriate therapy be employed when the pathogenic species is present and unnecessary treatment be avoided when it is not. It is important to remember, however, that it is by no means unusual to find *both* species present in the same individual. If a great many *E. coli* are present, it is easy to understand how a few cysts of *E. histolytica* may escape notice.

Trophozoites of *E. coli* are sluggishly motile in fresh, unstained preparations. The pseudopodia are relatively short and broad, and minimal locomotion is accomplished by their slow and apparently aimless activity. The cytoplasm appears rather coarse and viscid as compared to that of *E. histolytica,* and the pseudopodia are not hyaline as in the pathogenic species. In living specimens, the ectoplasm of *E. coli* is not clearly distinguishable from the endoplasm. Numerous food vacuoles, frequently containing ingested bacteria, are seen in the cytoplasm. Erythrocytes are very rarely ingested by this species; their presence should cause the examiner to suspect that the ameba is not *E. coli*. The nucleus is more likely to be visible in living trophozoites of *E. coli* than in those of *E. histolytica*. The nucleus appears as a ring of refractile granules surrounding the eccentrically placed karyosome. Despite the differential features enumerated, it is sometimes impossible to distinguish unstained trophozoites of *E. coli* from those of *E. histolytica*.

In preparations stained with iron hematoxylin, the single, rather large nucleus exhibits a heavy nuclear membrane lined by coarse, irregularly distributed granules, or plaques of chromatin. The karyosome is eccentrically placed and quite often is irregular in shape. Karyosomal chromatin is usually compact but may be dispersed. It is likely to be considerably heavier and more dense than the karyosome of *E. histolytica*. Chromatin particles are frequently seen between the karyosome and the nuclear membrane. The densely granular cytoplasm is commonly vacuolated, and ingested bacteria are often present. Red blood cells are not typically seen. A less granular, narrow rim of ectoplasm may sometimes be distinguished at the periphery of the organism. The trophozoites tend to be larger than those of *E. histolytica*, but they may be smaller.

SEE COLOR PLATE VIII FOR PHOTOMICROGRAPHS DEMONSTRATING THE TROPHOZOITES OF *Entamoeba coli.*

Cysts of *E. coli* are subject to pronounced variation in size. While generally larger than those of *E. histolytica*, they may be smaller. The unstained cysts seen in saline mounts display the usual highly refractile wall and less refractive cytoplasm, which is more densely granular than that of *E. histolytica*. The nuclei, one to eight in number, are easily visible in most instances. The eccentric position of the karyosome is often discernible, even in unstained preparations. Variation in refractility as compared to the surrounding cytoplasm may render chromatoidal bodies visible.

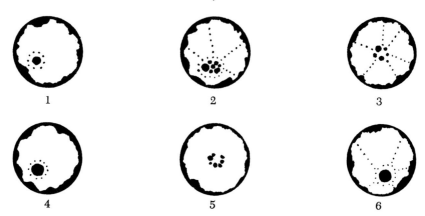

Diagram 2. Variations in nuclear morphology of *E. coli*: trophozoites (1, 4) and cysts (2, 3, 5, 6).

When stained with iodine, the cysts appear as yellow-brown, brightly refractile, spherical or ovoid bodies. Nuclei stand out clearly, and chromatoidals may occasionally be distinguished. Glycogen masses stain dark reddish brown if fresh material is used but may be a light yellowish brown color if the specimen has been concentrated by the formalin ether technique.

Permanent stains reveal the characteristic clear zone surrounding the cyst, which represents its unstained wall. Details of nuclear structure are demonstrated clearly in preparations stained with iron hematoxylin. The karyosome in uninucleate and binucleate cysts is apt to be composed of dense chromatin deposits, which are frequently dispersed in these young, actively dividing nuclei. The immature, active nucleus is usually large and may be elongate, ovoidal, or elliptical in shape, rather than spherical. Chromatin material lining the inner surface of the nuclear membrane is composed of dense, irregularly distributed granules arranged in aggregates or uneven plaques. Chromatin particles are quite often seen in the space between the karyosome and the nuclear membrane. As nuclear division proceeds to form the normal complement of eight nuclei, the individual nuclei become smaller, more delicate, and more perfectly spherical. Granules of chromatin lining the nuclear membrane in the mature cysts are quite small and are usually distributed evenly. Although the nuclear karyosome may be compact and punctiform, it is more likely to be composed of several small chromatin granules arranged in a semicircle or "horseshoe" pattern. The karyosome is usually eccentric in position but is centrally located with sufficient frequency to invalidate the widely held impression that this is a reliable and distinctive morphologic feature in the differential diagnosis between *E. coli* and *E. histolytica*. Diagram 2 depicts the nuclear detail of the cysts and trophozoites of *E. coli*.

Rarely, large cysts of *E. coli* will be observed that contain sixteen or more nuclei. These supernucleate forms are not, however, a problem in differential diagnosis. Diagnostic difficulty is encountered when the number of nuclei is four or less. In this connection it is helpful to keep in mind the distinction between the active nucleus and the nucleus in repose. If, for example, one or more of the four nuclei in a cyst exhibit evidence of karyokinetic activity, it may be assumed that further nuclear division will take place. In such cases the cyst will have eight nuclei when maturity is reached, and *E. histolytic* can be eliminated from consideration in the differential diagnosis.

Iron hematoxylin stained cysts of *E. coli* exhibit very coarse cytoplasmic granules, but these are usually much more evenly distributed than are the finer cytoplasmic granules of *E. histolytic cysts*. As a result, the alveolar, spongy appearance of the cytoplasm so common in cysts of *E. histolytica* is not seen in this species. Vacuoles, appearing as clear spaces in the cytoplasm, are frequently present in the stained cysts of *E. coli*. Very immature uninucleate or binucleate cysts may present a singular appearance due to the huge glycogen vacuoles that commonly occupy most of the body of the cysts. Such young forms regularly possess large nuclei showing evidence of karyokinetic activity, and numerous small chromatoidals are usually arranged around the margin of the cyst.

Chromatoidals are frequently found in the cysts of *E. coli*, though somewhat less often and less abundantly than in cysts of *E. histolytica*. The chromatoidal bodies often have jagged or splintered ends and are generally more irregular than those of the pathogenic species. Narrow, threadlike chromatoidals are not uncommon, and smoothly rounded or nearly spherical forms may be seen. As the cysts mature, chromatoidal bodies as well as glycogen vacuoles diminish in size and number. In ripe cysts containing eight nuclei, these cytoplasmic inclusions are frequently absent.

SEE COLOR PLATES IX, X, XI, AND XII FOR PHOTOMICROGRAPHS DEMONSTRATING THE CYSTS OF *Entamoeba coli.*

Entamoeba polecki

Entamoeba polecki is a widely distributed and common parasite in the intestine of pigs and monkeys. Available evidence does not indicate pathogenicity for man, although it has occasionally been identified in human feces since Kessel and Johnstone (1949) reported finding two human infections in California. The clinical importance of this ameba resides solely in the possibility of its being confused with *E. histolytica.*

Trophozoites of *E. polecki* so closely resemble those of *E. coli* that accurate differentiation is probably not possible, even in smears stained with iron hematoxylin. Motility of the trophozoites is sluggish and rarely directional. The granular and coarsely vacuolated cytoplasm often contains ingested bacteria. In permanent stains, the nuclear karyosome is usually seen to be centrally located and compact, but its chromatin is sometimes dispersed. Chromatin lining the nuclear membrane is quite often coarse and irregularly distributed, though in a few instances it is fine and evenly arranged.

Cysts of *E. polecki* are virtually always uninucleate. Binucleate cysts have rarely been observed. In cysts stained with iron hematoxylin, deposits of nuclear chromatin are likely to be heavy and evenly distributed along the nuclear membrane. Nuclear chromatin in some cysts appears as a regularly arranged layer of delicately beaded granules and in others as an aggregate of coarse chromatin forming uneven plaques. The karyosome is centrally located in a majority of cysts but occasionally is eccentric. Karyosomal chromatin is usually dispersed, but it may be compact.

Abundant chromatoidals, many being rod shaped, with pointed or angular ends, are likely to be present in cysts of this species. A few chromatoidals having smooth and rounded ends are encountered. Chromatoidal bodies are frequently small, and spherical, threadlike, and irregularly shaped forms may be seen.

A unique morphologic feature found in more than half of the cysts of *E. polecki* is the "inclusion mass." This ill-defined spherical or ovoid mass stains uniformly with iron hematoxylin, though much less intensely than the chromatoidals or nuclear structures. Its nature is unknown, but it is believed not to be glycogen, since it is not dissolved out to leave a clear space in the iron hematoxylin stained smears, and it does not stain characteristically with iodine in the wet mounts. When present, this distinctive inclusion mass provides a reliable means of identifying *E. polecki*. Because of it, and the exclusively uninucleate character of cysts, differentiation from *E. histolytica* is not difficult.

SEE COLOR PLATE **XII** FOR PHOTOMICROGRAPHS DEMONSTRATING THE TROPHOZOITES AND CYSTS OF *Entamoeba polecki.*

Iodamoeba bütschlii

Iodamoeba bütschlii is a nonpathogenic intestinal ameba found throughout the world, though it is less common than *E. coli* or *E. nana*. It is to be distinguished from the pathogenic species. This is ordinarily not difficult, even in the saline and iodine mounts, and is quite easy when the iron hematoxyline stain is utlized.

Trophozoites of *Iodamoeba bütschlii* display exceptional variations in size, overlapping the size range of the pathogenic species as well as that of the small nonpathogenic amebae. The trophozoites are sluggishly motile, occasionally achieving limited progressive movement. The very granular and diffusely vacuolated cytoplasm usually contains ingested bacteria. Yeasts, detritus, and other food inclusions may be seen at times. Red blood cells are not ingested. The clear ectoplasm is not readily distinguishable from the densely granular endoplasm, but hyaline pseudopodia are sometimes visible.

The single nucleus is recognized with some difficulty in living specimens. Details of nuclear structure become visible in smears stained with iron hematoxylin or the trichrome stain. The large, irregularly rounded nuclear karyosome appears to be contained in a vacuole, since the delicate nuclear membrane usually does not take the stain and remains invisible. The karyosome may be either central or eccentric in position. A layer of tiny granules surrounding the karyosome is visible only under optimal conditions and can rarely be distinguished.

Cysts of *I. bütschlii* are commonly ovoidal or irregularly pyriform in shape but may be spherical. They are quite distinctive in preparations stained with iodine, due to the unfailing presence of a large, sharply-outlined, and exceptionally dense glycogen vacuole. In fresh material, iodine stains the ovoidal, polygonal, or irregularly spherical glycogen mass a deep reddish brown. In older, fixed, or concentrated specimens, the glycogen is likely to stain less deeply and may be yellow or yellow-brown in color. The nucleus with its large karyosome may be visible as a highly refractile structure within the cytoplasm.

The large glycogen vacuole, which may occupy nearly half of the cyst, is seen as a characteristic, sharply defined clear space in the iron hematoxylin stains. The distinctive nuclear structure of the cysts of this species, as seen in the permanent stains, makes confusion with any other amebic cyst most unlikely. The rather large, often irregularly shaped nuclear karyosome is usually eccentric in position. The delicate, unstained nuclear membrane is devoid of peripheral chromatin and remains invisible. In the majority of cysts an aggregate of chromatin granules is interposed between the karyosome and the nuclear membrane. These granules are usually arranged in the form of a crescent, partially surrounding the nuclear karyosome. At times they are minute and delicate, so that individual granules are easily distinguishable. Often the chromatin granules form a coarse aggregate, which may be crescentic, roughly triangular, or irregularly oval in shape. To some observers the resulting appearance has suggested a "basket of flowers"; others may visualize a "cap," perched upon the nuclear karyosome. In occasional instances no chromatin granules are visible in the space between the karyosome and the nuclear membrane. In these cysts, when the karyosome is centrally located, the nuclear structure may be indistinguishable from that of the trophozoites. Binucleate cysts have rarely been reported. Diagram 3 demonstrates the nuclear detail of the cysts and trophozoites of *I. bütschlii*.

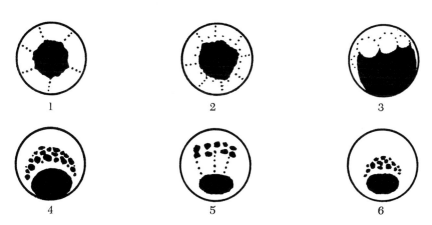

Diagram 3. Variations in nuclear morphology of *I. bütschlii*: trophozoites (1, 2) and cysts (3 through 6).

SEE COLOR PLATES **XIII** AND **XIV** FOR PHOTOMICROGRAPHS DEMONSTRATING THE TROPHOZOITES AND CYSTS OF *Iodamoeba bütschlii.*

Endolimax nana

Endolimax nana is a cosmopolitan and extremely common intestinal parasite, being found even more frequently than *E. coli* in some populations. One of the smaller amebae, it is harmless to man and produces no clinical symptoms. Its importance lies in the fact that difficulty may be experienced in differentiating both the cysts and trophozoites from those of the small race of *E. histolytica*.

Trophozoites of *E. nana* are approximately the same size as its cysts, though the cystic forms display even greater variations in size. The trophozoites are sluggishly motile, through the

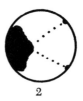

1   2   3

Diagram 4. Variations in nuclear morphology of *E. nana*; trophozoites (1) and cysts (2, 3).

action of short, blunt hyaline pseudopodia. Progressive and directional movement is not commonly seen, although active trophozoites found in freshly passed liquid stools may accomplish some locomotion. The cytoplasm is finely granular and vacuolated. Ingested bacteria are usually present. The nucleus is not often visible in the unstained trophozoites.

In fecal smears stained with iron hematoxylin, the characteristic nuclear structure may be studied. The small spherical or subspherical nucleus contains a large and prominent karyosome, which may be centrally placed, but it is somewhat more frequently eccentric in location. The karyosome may be smooth and rounded, lobulated, or quite irregular in shape. The nuclear membrane is not furnished with peripheral chromatin, though it is likely to be heavier and more easily distinguished than is that of *I. bütschlii*. The details of nuclear structure and the appearance of the cytoplasm of trophozoites of *E. nana* so closely resemble those of *I. bütschlii* that accurate differentiation of the two species may be extremely difficult.

Cysts of *E. nana* are most frequently ovoidal in shape; however, spherical and subspherical forms are occasionally seen. The usual refractile cyst wall is present and is best seen in wet mounts stained with iodine. Little detail is visible in either the unstained or iodine-stained preparations, though the nuclei can generally be distinguished. Glycogen masses may be present in the cytoplasm but are usually diffuse and poorly defined.

In fecal smears stained with iron hematoxylin the cysts are seen to possess one to four nuclei, the mature quadrinucleate cyst being the most commonly found. The nuclear structure is characterized by a large and frequently irregular karyosome that is usually eccentric in position. The nuclear membrane lacks deposits of chromatin and may not be easily visible. Infrequently, tiny, slightly curved chromatoidal rods are seen in the cytoplasm. Diagram 4 shows the nuclear detail of the cysts and trophozoites of *E. nana*.

SEE COLOR PLATE XV FOR PHOTOMICROGRAPHS DEMONSTRATING THE TROPHOZITES AND CYSTS OF *Endolimax nana.*

Dientamoeba fragilis

Dientamoeba fragilis is not a common species but has been found throughout the world wherever a diligent search has been made. The exact taxonomic position of *D. fragilis* is in doubt, and several prominent investigators believe that morpholigic features place it as a relative of the ameba-flagellate *Histomonas meleagridis*, a common parasite of turkeys and other domestic birds. Despite this suspicion, flagella have never been demonstrated in the trophozoites of *D. fragilis*. Furthermore, a cystic stage of this protozoan is not recognized, and the method of transmission is uncertain. While this small ameba is not known to invade or destroy tissue, it seems certain that it is capable of producing abdominal discomfort and a troublesome diarrhea.

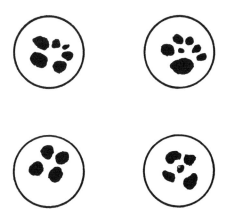

Diagram 5. Variations in nuclear morphology of *D. fragilis*.

Trophozoites of *D. fragilis* are unique, in that they characteristically possess two nuclei. This binucleate structure, found in more than three fourths of the organisms, serves to distinguish them from all other amebic trophozoites that infect man. The trophozoites exhibit considerable variation but are generally about the same size as those of *E. nana*. Motility is active, and progressive movement may be seen. The broad and sometimes serrated pseudopodia are distinctly hyaline. The ectoplasm is usually quite clearly distinguishable from the endoplasm. In hematoxylin-stained fecal smears, the cytoplasm is observed to be heavily vacuolated, and ingested bacteria are often present.

The nuclei of *D. fragilis* are invisible when unstained but exhibit characteristic and unique structure when stained with iron hematoxylin. The delicate nuclear membrane is devoid of peripheral chromatin granules and may not be clearly seen. The karyosome is composed of from four to eight separate chromatin granules, which are usually located in the center of the nucleus. The individual granules may be seen clearly in well-stained preparations and are typically arranged in a symmetrical fashion. A rosette or tetrad arrangement is most common, but a variety of irregular patterns and bandlike clusters of chromatin granules may be noted. The presence of a preponderance of binucleate forms provides an adequate basis for accurate species identification, when taken together with the distinctive nuclear morphology demonstrated in the iron hematoxylin stained slides. Diagram 5 depicts the nuclear detail of the trophozoites of *D. fragilis*.

SEE COLOR PLATE XVI FOR PHOTOMICROGRAPHS DEMONSTRATING THE TROPHOZOITES OF *Dientamoeba fragilis*.

Entamoeba gingivalis

Entamoeba gingivalis, while not a true intestinal ameba, deserves brief mention here. This prevalent parasite is a commensal in the oral cavity of man, thriving in the presence of gingival inflammation, pyorrhea alveolaris, or diseased tonsils. It may rarely appear in the sputum, where its presence may cause confusion due to the pronounced morphologic similarity of this species to *E. histolytica*. Under these circumstances, an erroneous diagnosis of pulmonary abscess due to *E. histolytica* may be made.

Trophozoites of *E. gingivalis* possess a single nucleus, which is not distinguishable morphologically from that of *E. histolytica*. The vacuolated cytoplasm, however, contains ingested bacteria and nuclear fragments of partly digested leucocytes, but rarely erythrocytes. The easily recognizable fragments of ingested leucocytes serve to identify *E. gingivalis*, for other species do not ingest these cells. A cyst stage of this species is not known.

SEE COLOR PLATE I, FIG 3, FOR A PHOTOMICROGRAPH SHOWING THE TROPHOZOITES OF *Entamoeba gingivalis.*

THE FLAGELLATES

Giardia lamblia

Giardia lamblia is the only intestinal flagellate that is capable of inducing symptoms. While it is sometimes a harmless commensal, clinical observations document diarrhea, vague abdominal complaints, intestinal malabsorption, and immunodeficiency states as being associated with giardiasis. This cosmopolitan flagellate is one of the most commonly encountered intestinal protozoan parasites, and it is probable that animal vectors, such as beavers, dogs, muskrats, and others, play a role in contaminating water with infectious cysts.

Trophozoites of *G. lamblia* exhibit rapid, erratic, irregularly progressive motility that is rather distinctive. Only when cooling or other environmental factors have slowed the organisms nearly to a halt is it possible to distinguish some of the flagella and the general morphology. The bilaterally symmetrical trophozoite is rounded at the anterior end and sharply tapered posteriorly. Two nuclei, one situated on each side of the midline in the anterior one third of the organism, can be demonstrated in the permanently stained smears. The rather large ovoidal nuclei possess a delicate nuclear membrane which lacks peripheral chromatin. The nuclear karyosome may be dense and compact or may consist of a well-dispersed mass of small chromatin granules. It is usually central in position. The four pairs of flagella do not stain well with iron hematoxylin or the trichrome stain and usually remain invisible. The two nuclei are located in the area of the ventral sucking disk, which occupies most of the anterior half of the organism. Immediately posterior to this disk, lying transversely across the midline, are the median bodies. They appear as closely placed, heavy, slightly curved rods that are aptly described as "claw-hammer" in appearance. The median bodies are important differential morphologic features in the separation of *Giardia lamblia* from other species of *Giardia* encountered in lower animals. The intracytoplasmic portions of the flagella, called the axonemes, can be distinguished in part.

Cysts of *Giardia* are regularly ovoidal objects easily recognized by the characteristic shape, highly refractile, delicate cyst wall, finely granular cytoplasm, nuclei, and intracytoplasmic flagellar structures. These morphologic features may be partly visualized in unstained preparations but are better demonstrated after staining with iodine. Additional detail is brought out in the fecal smears stained with iron hematoxylin or the trichrome stain. Two nuclei are present in the recently formed cysts, and four nuclei are found in mature cysts. The dense, compact nuclear karyosomes may be either central or eccentric in position. The delicate and usually invisible nuclear membrane is not furnished with peripheral chromatin. Curved fragments of the ventral sucking disk can usually be identified, as well as intracytoplasmic extensions of the flagella, the axonemes, which are dispersed in four paired groups. Due to shrinkage of the cytoplasm at the time of fixation, the fine cytoplasm is quite often separated from the cyst wall in permanent stains. However, this phenomenon is also observed frequently in fresh, unstained preparations.

SEE COLOR PLATE XVII FOR PHOTOMICROGRAPHS DEMONSTRATING THE TROPHOZOITES AND CYSTS OF *Giardia lamblia.*

Chilomastix mesnili

Chilomastix mesnili is a nonpathogenic flagellate widely distributed throughout the world but more prevalent in warm climates. It lives as a harmless commensal in the intestine of man and is believed not to be responsible for any clinical symptoms. It must be distinguished from *Giardia lamblia* and the other flagellate protozoa occasionally found in fecal specimens.

Trophozoites of *C. mesnili* are rounded anteriorly, tapered posteriorly, and are marked by a spiral groove through the middle half of the body. Living specimens exhibit active and progressive motility that is jerky and irregular, as is usual with the flagellate protozoa. The three anterior flagella are easily distinguished in fresh preparation but rarely stain well enough to be visible at the iron hematoxylin stains.

In the permanently stained smears, a single spherical nucleus is seen near the anterior pole of the organism. A small, central karyosome is usually, but not always, present. Plaques of chromatin are often seen on the inner surface of the nuclear membrane. The elongate cytostome is usually visible beside the nucleus, or partly obscured by it. The cytostomal fibrils curve posteriorly around the cytostome. The cytoplasm of the trophozoite is delicately granular and diffusely vacuolated.

Cysts of *C. mesnili*, in saline and iodine mounts as well as in smears stained with iron hematoxylin, are quite readily recognized on the basis of their distinctive shape and thick cyst wall. Due to the conspicuous nipple-like prominence, the cyst has a characteristic pear-shaped or lemon-shaped appearance. The dense cytoplasm is often retracted from the narrower end of the cyst. Smears stained with iron hematoxylin demonstrate a single nucleus with a large and frequently irregular karyosome, which may be either central or eccentric in position. Cytostomal fibrils may be visible.

SEE COLOR PLATE XVIII FOR PHOTOMICROGRAPHS DEMONSTRATING THE TROPHOZOITES AND CYSTS OF *Chilomastix mesnili.*

Trichomonas hominis

Trichomonas hominis is generally believed to be a harmless commensal in the digestive tract of man, but occasional presence in diarrheic stools has caused some speculation regarding its ability to induce clinical symptoms. This cosmopolitan intestinal flagellate is nearly as prevalent as *Giardia*. Since a cyst stage for this organism is not known, it is believed that infection of *Trichomonas* is indicative of direct fecal contamination.

Trophozoites of *Trichomonas* exhibit jerky, rapid, and erratic motility, which is progressive but not directional. When motility has been sufficiently slowed by environmental factors, it is possible to distinguish four or five anterior flagella. An undulating membrane extends posteriorly along the pyriform body of the organism, its free margin marked by a recurrent flagellum with a free trailing end. The characteristic wavelike motion of the undulating membrane is distinctive and easily recognized. The sharp posterior end of the semirigid axostyle may be seen to extend through the cytoplasm, forming the pointed terminal end of the tapered body.

Difficulty may be experienced in staining this species with iron hematoxylin, and in such preparations the flagella and the undulating membrane are poorly seen. The costa, a relatively thick, curved rod marking the attachment of the undulating membrane, stains well and is a useful diagnostic feature. The single nucleus, located at the anterior end of the flagellate, is furnished with a conspicuous central karyosome. Fine chromatin granules may line the nuclear membrane.

SEE COLOR PLATE **XVIII** FOR A PHOTOMICROGRAPH DEMONSTRATING THE TROPHOZOITE OF *Trichomonas hominis.*

THE COCCIDIA

Isospara belli and *Isospora hominis*

Isospora belli has been widely confused with *Isospora*

hominis until quite recently, and many examiners continue to make this common error in species identification. The careful descriptions of Elsdon-Dew and his associates (1953) clarify the distinction between the two species and should prevent such mistakes from continuing. Both members of the genus *Isospora* belong to the subphylum Sporozoa, the subclass Coccidia, and the order Eimeriidea; but *I. belli* is the species that is usually recognized. *I. hominis* is much less common and is very rarely discovered in direct fecal films. Infections with *Isospora* are now known to be more common than was formerly suspected. Available evidence indicates that definite gastrointestinal symptoms, including severe diarrhea and fatal malabsorption, may in some instances result from infection with *Isospora*.

All stages in the development of the oocyst of *I. belli* may be found in the stool. The immature oocysts are colorless, double-walled, highly refractile, ellipsoidal or ovoidal bodies, containing a spherical mass of very granular protoplasm. The protoplasmic mass within the oocyst soon divides, forming two sporoblasts, each of which then secretes a heavy cyst wall. Within each daughter spore, now called a sporocyst, further division takes place to form four sausage-shaped sporozoites. These curved, crescentic bodies can be readily distinguished from the granular mass of sporocystic residue. After breaking out of the oocystic membrane, the two sporocysts of *I. belli*, each containing four sporozoites, are rarely discovered in the feces.

Isospora hominis, unlike *I. belli,* is typically mature when passed in the feces, the sporocysts having already escaped from the oocystic membrane. The sporocysts may be seen singly, or occasionally in adherent pairs. Rarely is any vestige of the oocystic membrane visible. Thus, it can be understood how the sporocysts of *I. hominis,* much smaller than the oocysts of *I. belli* and lacking the refractile outer oocyst wall, usually escape detection on routine stool examinations.

SEE COLOR PLATE **XIX** FOR PHOTOMICROGRAPHS DEMONSTRATING THE OOCYSTS OF *Isospora belli.*

Eimeria stiedae

Eimeria stiedae is a common parasite of rabbits, which has, in a few instances, been suspected of causing disease in man. It is probable, however, that this species is a spurious parasite of man. Several related members of the genus *Eimeria* have been found, now and then, in human feces, but it is generally agreed that they are pseudoparasites "in transit," as a result of ingestion of the tissues of their natural host.

E. stiedae can easily be distinguished from the closely related members of the genus *Isospora* by its larger size, and by the fact that its mature oocysts contain four sporocysts, in contrast to the two present in mature oocysts of *Isospora*. Each sporocyst of *Eimeria* contains two sporozoites, instead of the four found in each sporocyst of *Isospora*.

E. stiedae is much larger than either *I. belli* or *I. hominis*, approximating in size some of the smaller helminth eggs. *Because of this, the photomicrographs demonstrating this species had to be made at the lower magnification otherwise reserved for the helminth eggs.*

SEE COLOR PLATE **XX** FOR PHOTOMICROGRAPHS DEMONSTRATING THE OOCYSTS OF *Eimeria stiedae*.

THE CILIATES

Balantidium coli

Balantidium coli has the distinction of being the only member of the class Ciliatea known to parasitize man. There are a number of free-living and coprozoic species among the ciliate protozoa that resemble *B. coli*, and those must be distinguished from the pathogenic species. *B. coli* of man is indistinguishable morphologically from *B. coli* var. *suis*, which is found commonly in domestic hogs, but man is usually quite refractory to infection with the porcine variety.

B. coli is known to be a tissue invader and is capable of producing severe ulcerative lesions of the intestinal mucosa; in very rare instances it can mestastasize to distant organs. While some persons infected with this parasite will be asymptomatic, a majority will experience diarrhea; and some will develop severe dysentery with accompanying abdominal cramping pain and generalized complaints. Infections with *B. coli* are not common, but when environmental circumstances favor its dissemination, balantidiasis may occur in epidemic form

B. coli is the largest protozoan species parasitizing man, and it may nearly be visible to the unaided eye. There is considerable variation in the size of the trophozoites, but average organisms approximate the common helminth eggs in size. *For this reason, in making the photomicrographs that demonstrate this species, it was necessary to utlize the lower magnification ordinarily reserved for the helminth eggs.*

Trophozoites of *B. coli* are large, ovoidal bodies covered with short cilia, whose vigorous and synchronized motion rapidly propels the organism in purposeful but erratic fashion. The cytostome is located near the more pointed anterior end of the ciliate, somewhat toward its flattened side. This slightly curved, funnel-shaped depression is lined with long and heavy cilia. Numerous food vacuoles may be seen in the cytoplasm. The large macronucleus may be visible in unstained preparations, but it is more distinctly seen when the organism has been stained with iodine. Additional details are brought out in smears stained with iron hematoxylin. The macronucleus is usually elongate and bean shaped, but may be ovoidal, spherical, or kidney shaped. For the most part it is eccentrically located near the middle of the body and appears as a solid and dense mass of chromatin in slides stained with iron hematoxylin. The tiny micronucleus may be seen as a compact, punctiform mass of dense chromatin, located adjacent ot the inner curvature of the macronucleus. It may be hidden by the larger nucleus.

Cysts of *B. coli* are spherical or ellipsoidal bodies, about half the size of the trophozoites. The rounded cysts possess a thick, refractile wall. Cilia can sometimes be distinguished if the organism is newly encysted. The macronucleus and large cytoplasmic vacuoles are visible in stained specimens, but other structures are not readily recognized.

SEE COLOR PLATE **XX** FOR PHOTOMICROGRAPHS DEMONSTRATING THE TROPHOZOITES AND CYSTS *Balantidium coli.*

COLOR ATLAS

Color Plate I

Figure 1. Polymorphonuclear leucocytes. These familial cells may be used as a standard for visual size comparison. Refer back to this photomicrograph when studying the size and morphology of the various protozan parasite forms and pseudoparasites shown in Color Plates I through XIX. Iron hemagoxylin stain.

Figure 2. This large mononuclear phagocyte has ingested a polymorphonuclear leucocyte. Compare with the trophozoites of *Entamoeba histolytica* shown in Color Plates I and II. This pseudoparasite is from the stool of a patient having idiopathic ulcerative colitis. Iron hematoxylin stain.

Figure 3. *Entamoeba gingivalis* (trophozoite). This harmless commensal closely resembles *Entamoeba histolytica*. It may be found in the sputum, where it could be mistaken for *E. histolytica* from a pulmonary abscess. Note the typical *Entamoeba* nucleus. The nuclear fragments of ingested leucocytes serve to distinguish the two species. Iron hematoxylin stain.

Figure 4. *Entamoeba histolytica* (trophozoite), from the stool of a patient with acute amebic dysentery. Notice the presence of numerous ingested erythrocytes, which partially surround the delicate nucleus. Iron hematoxylin stain.

Figure 5. This phagocytic structure was found in the stool of a patient having bacillary dysentery. Comparison with Figures 4 and 6 will demonstrate how a careless or inexperienced examiner might confuse such a degenerated cellular structure with an amebic tropozoite. Iron hematoxylin stain.

Figure 6. *Entamoeba histolytica* (trophozoite). Notice particularly the delicate nuclear structure and the central position of the karyosome. Four ingested erythrocytes in various stages of digestion are seen in the cytoplasm. Iron hematoxylin.

Figure 7. This trophozoite of *Entamoeba histolytica* exhibits characteristic nuclear structure and cytoplasm with several small pseudopods. The cytoplasm contains ingested erythrocytes but no bacteria or other debris. Iron hematoxylin stain.

Figure 8. The small trophozoite of *Entamoeba histolytica* shown in this photomicrograph has not ingested red blood cells. The delicate nucleus with a centrally placed punctate karyosome is typical. Notice that the endoplasm is sharply delimited from the ectoplasm of the pseudopods. Iron hematoxylin stain.

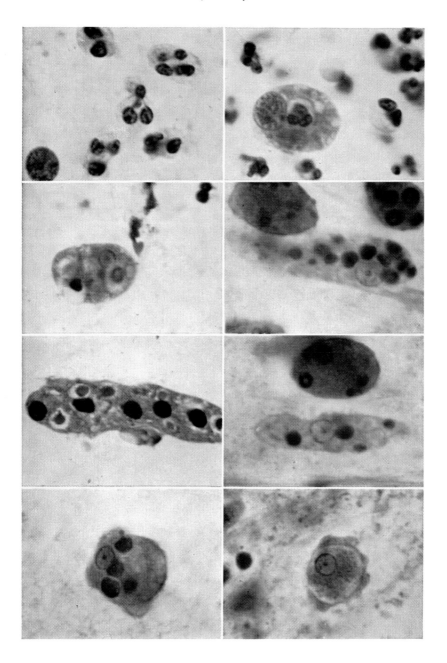

Color Plate II

Figure 1. Fragments of several ingested red blood cells are present in the cytoplasm of this slightly degenerate trophozoite of *Entamoeba histolytica*. Chromatin material lining the nuclear membrane is unusually heavy for the trophozoites of this species. Iron hematoxylin stain.

Figure 2. *Entamoeba histolytica* (trophozoite). Again the chromatin material lining the inner surface of the nuclear membrane is somewhat heavier than is usual for this species. No erythrocytes have been ingested. Iron hematoxylin stain.

Figure 3. This large trophozoite of *Entamoeba histolytica* has ingested more than a dozen red blood cells. The lightly stained nucleus is somewhat distorted but can be recognized at the lower margin of the trophozoite. Iron hematoxylin stain.

Figure 4. *Entamoeba histolytica* (trophozoite). Several ingested erythrocytes are present in the cytoplasm. Notice that the nuclear karyosome is slightly eccentric in position. This is rather unusual in the trophozoites of this species. Trichrome stain.

Figure 5. *Entamoeba histolytica* (trophozoite). The nuclear structure seen in this photomicrograph is entirely typical of the trophozoites of this species. A single ingested erythrocyte is present in the cytoplasm. Trichrome stain.

Figure 6. *Entamoeba histolytica* (trophozoite). Again the nuclear karyosome is seen to lie in an eccentric position. The trophozoite is otherwise morphologically characteristic for this species. Trichrome stain.

Figure 7(a). *Entamoeba histolytica* (trophozoite). The very typical and perfect *Entamoeba* nucleus (lower right) is well shown in this place of optical focus. Trichrome stain.

Figure 7(b). The same trophozoite of *Entamoeba histolytica* is shown at a lower level of optical focus in this photomicrograph. The pseudopodia and the fragments of ingested red blood cells are better demonstrated, but the nucleus is not visible in this focal plane.

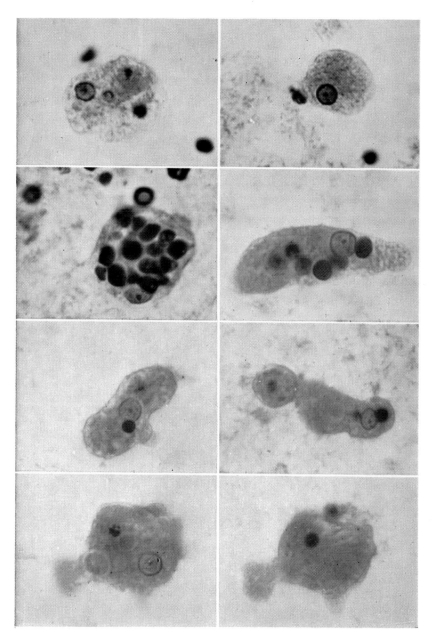

Color Plate III

Figure 1. A trophozite of *Entamoeba histolytica* is shown here projecting several pseudopods. The nucleus is clearly seen in this unstained specimen; however, a permanent stain is necessary to accurately determine morphology. The trophozoites shown here and above were from an axenic culture of *E. histolytica*.

Figure 2. A large unstained motile trophozoite of *Entamoeba histolytica*. Note the clear, hyaline-appearing pseudopod extruding from the right superior aspect of the organism. Somewhat below, the nucleus is clearly seen as a rounded collection of dots.

Figure 3. A trophozoite of *Entamoeba histolytica* packed with engulfed erythrocytes. The identification of erythrocytes within the endoplasm is an important diagnostic point, inasmuch as nonpathogenic species seldom, if ever, exhibit this feature.

Figure 4. This photomicrograph, taken a few seconds later, demonstrates a rapid change in configuration as the trophozoites move.

Figure 5. An actively motile hematophageous trophozoite. The nucleus is faintly visible as a series of dots and is located in the right midportion of the protozoan.

Figure 6. The same trophozoite photographed a few seconds later and exhibiting rapid motility.

Figure 7. A trophozoite of *Entamoeba histolytica* (unstained) in the process of ingesting red blood cells. Note the enveloping of the red cell by the ameba.

Figure 8. An earlier photograph of the same trophozoite. The nucleus can be seen faintly below the erythrocyte.

(X1320)

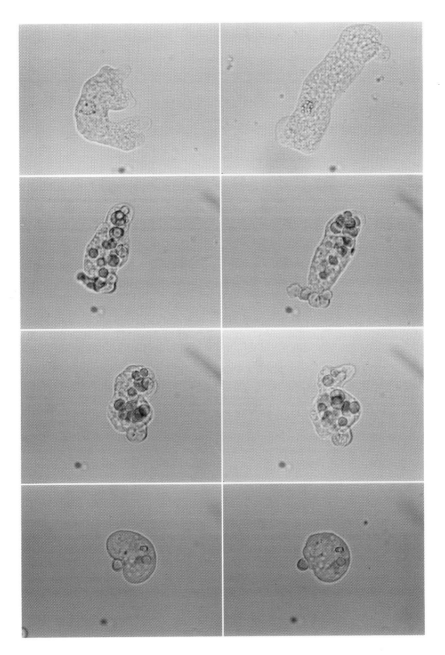

Color Plate IV

Figure 1. *Entamoeba histolytica* (large race, cyst). The large chromatoidal bar with smooth and rounded ends is the type most often found in the cysts of this species. A single small, resting nucleus is seen at the upper margin of the cysts. Three additonal nuclei present in this mature cyst are not visible in this focal plane. Iron hematoxylin stain.

Figure 2. *Entamoeba histolytica* (large race). The chromatoidal body in this cyst is irregularly shaped, and the two nuclei visible here show rather heavy chromatin material lining the nuclear membrane. The nuclear karyosomes are eccentrically placed. Iron hematoxylin stain.

Figure 3. *Entamoeba histolytica* (small race). This immature cyst contains a single nucleus with typically delicate structure, and a compact, very slightly eccentric karyosome. The finely granular cytoplasm is evenly distributed here, in contrast to the usual vacuolated pattern seen in the more mature cysts of this species. Iron hematoxylin stain.

Figure 4. This mature cyst of *Entamoeba histolytica* (large race) contains four resting nuclei, which are seen in sharp or partial focus in this photomicrograph. Three of the nuclei lie immediately adjacent to the narrow, irregularly shaped chromatoidal body. Iron hematoxylin stain.

Figure 5(a). *Entamoeba histolytica* (large race, cyst.). At this upper level of optical focus two of the four nuclei present in this mature cyst are visible, the one on the left being partially obscured by the shadow of an imperfectly focused chromatoidal body. Iron hematoxylin stain.

Figure 5(b). The same cyst as in Figure 5(a) is shown here in a lower focal plane, demonstrating the two additional nuclei present in this mature cyst of *Entamoeba histolytica*. Notice the characteristically central position of the nuclear karyosomes. The smooth, ovoidal chromatoidal body is now sharply focused.

Figure 6. *Entamoeba histolytica* (large race). This immature cyst contains a large glycogen vacuole and a heavy, irregularly shaped chromatoidal body, which lies adjacent to and partially surrounds the single nucleus. The diffuse karyosome and coarse nuclear chromatin are evidence of karyokinetic activity. Iron hematoxylin stain.

Figure 7. *Entamoeba histolytic* (large race). The two nuclei present in this cyst exhibit centrally placed karyosomes and uniform distribution of chromatin granules on the inner surface of the nuclear membrane, features that are characteristic of this species. Several narrow, irregularly shaped chromatoidal bars are present. Iron hematoxylin stain.

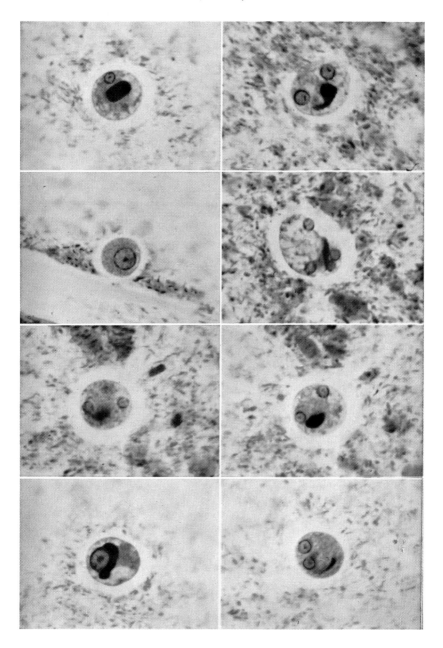

Color Plate V

Figure 1. *Entamoeba histolytica* (large race). Notice the diffuse arrangement of karyosomal chromatin in the active nucleus of this young cyst. Several small chromatoidal bodies lie adjacent to the delicate nucleus. A large glycogen vacuole is present. Trichrome stain.

Figure 2. *Entamoeba histolytica* (large race). Note the eccentric position of the nuclear karyosome in this young cyst. The karyosome is not always central in position in the cysts of this species. The ovoidal chromatoidal body is a bright pink color in this preparation stained with the trichrome stain.

Figure 3. *Entamoeba histolytica* (large race). Numerous small chromatoidals are seen surrounding the large glycogen vacuole in this very young, uninucleate cyst. The elongate, ovoid nucleus with diffuse karyosomal structure denotes karyokinetic activity. Such immature cysts may confuse an inexperienced examiner. Iron hematoxylin stain.

Figure 4. *Entamoeba histolytica* (large race). The cytoplasmic granules are typically fine but irregularly distributed in this young, uninucleate cyst. The nuclear chromatin is heavy, and the karyosome is coarse but rather compact. The chromatoidal body is unusually irregular in shape. Iron hematoxylin stain.

Figure 5. This photomicrograph demonstrates an iodine-stained cyst of *Entamoeba histolytica* (large race). The single nucleus demonstrates typically delicate structure. A chromatoidal body is visible above the nucleus.

Figure 6. *Entamoeba histolytica* (large race). Three of the four nuclei present in this iodine-stained cyst are visible in this focal plane. The cytoplasmic structure of this mature cyst is quite typical. Notice also the highly refractile cyst wall.

Figure 7. This iodine-stained cyst of *Entamoeba histolytica* is intermediate in size between the large and small races. Four nuclei are visible, arranged on each side of the chromatoidal body in the center of the cyst. Only the two nuclei at left are in sharp focus here, and in both the nuclear karyosome is eccentric in position.

Figure 8. This photomicrograph demonstrates an unstained cyst of *Entaomeba histolytica* (large race). One delicate, resting nucleus is present, having a punctate, central karyosome. A smooth, ovoidal chromatoidal bar occupies the lower portion of the cyst.

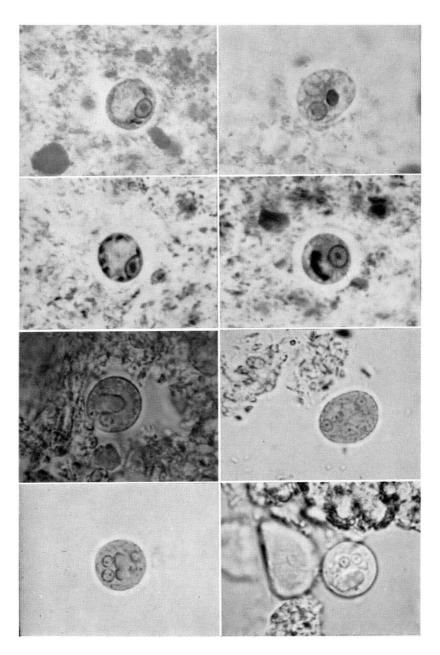

Color Plate VI

Figure 1. The delicately granular cytoplasm, smooth and ovoidal chromatoidal bars, and central position of the compact nuclear karyosome are all typical in this cyst of *Entamoeba histolytica*. The cyst is intermediate in size between the definitely small and obviously large races, as are several others on this Plate. Iron hematoxylin stain.

Figure 2. *Entamoeba histolytica* (large race). This young, uninucleate cyst contains a large, irregularly shaped glycogen vacuole and several small chromatoidal bodies. It is not uncommon for such young cysts to stain very deeply with the iron hematoxylin.

Figure 3(a). This mature cyst of *Entamoeba histolytica* is shown at an upper level of optical focus, demonstrating the presence of two of its four nuclei and a heavy chromatoidal bar with smooth and rounded ends. Iron hematoxylin stain.

Figure 3(b). The same cyst of *Entamoeba histolytica* as in Figure 3(a), photographed at a lower optical level, is shown in this photomicrograph. One additional nucleus has been brought into sharp focus. Notice the irregular distribution of fine granules, which results in the usual alveolar appearance of the cytoplasm.

Figure 4. This cyst of *Entamoeba histolytica* is also intermediate in size between the very small and the very large races of this species. It was obtained from an asymptomatic individual with no evidence of disease. Compare size with Figure 2, Plate V, with Figures 2 and 4, Plate IV, and with Figures 1 and 7, Plate VII. Iron hematoxylin stain.

Figure 5. This immature cyst of *Entamoeba histolytica* contains a large glycogen vacuole and a single nucleus showing karyokinetic activity. A small chromatoidal is seen adjacent to the nucleus. It is sometimes impossible to differentiate such young cysts as this one (and the one shown in Fig. 6) from those of *Entamoeba coli*. Iron hematoxylin stain.

Figure 6. *Entamoeba histolytica* (large race). The body of this young cyst is largely occupied by a glycogen vacuole, around which are arranged numerous small chromatoidal bars. The cyst is binucleate, the second kinetic nucleus lying below the focal plane in which this photomicrograph was made. Iron hematoxylin stain.

Figure 7. This mature cyst of *Entamoeba histolytica* contains four resting nuclei, two of which are hidden by the heavy chromatoidal body in this photomicrograph. Iron hematoxylin stain.

66

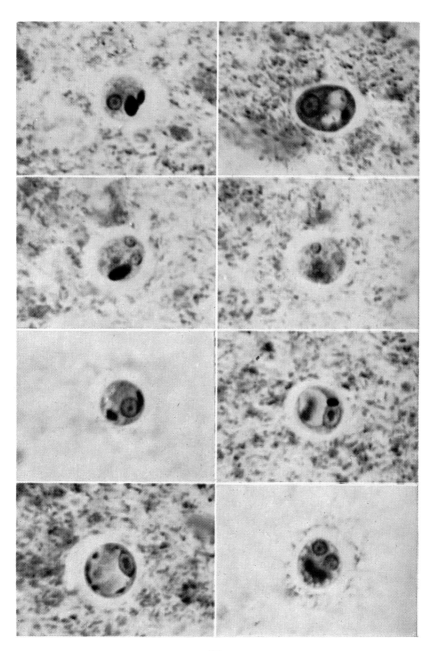

Color Plate VII

Figure 1. *Entamoeba histolytica* (small race). This very small, uninucleate cyst exhibits very fine cytoplasmic granules and a single smooth chromatoidal bar. The large nuclear karyosome appears heavy and coarse, and is actually composed of several small, closely grouped chromatin granules. Iron hematoxylin stain.

Figure 2. The cytoplasm of this cyst of *Entamoeba histolytica* shows the finely granular structure usually seen in this species. The chromatoidal body is unusually irregular in shape. The single delicate nucleus is quite typical of this species. Iron hematoxylin stain.

Figure 3. This immature cyst of *Entamoeba histolytica* (large race) possesses a large glycogen vacuole and a single ovoidal chromatoidal body that is a bright pink color in this trichrome-stained preparation. The diffuse karysomal structure denotes karyokinetic activity, as does the elongate, oval shape of the nucleus.

Figure 4. *Entamoeba histolytica* (large race). The cytoplasmic structure is quite typical, and several small chromatoidals are present in this immature cyst. The single large resting nucleus demonstrates characteristically delicate arrangement of chromatin and a tiny, punctate central karyosome. Trichrome stain.

Figure 5. *Entamoeba histolytica* (large race). Three mature resting nuclei are seen, together with a large and regularly shaped chromatoidal bar, which appears reddish pink in this preparation stained with the trichrome stain.

Figure 6. *Entamoeba histolytica* (large race). The vacuolated structure and alveolar, spongy appearance of the cytoplasm is common in the more mature cysts of this species and is quite distinctive, being rarely seen in the cysts of *Entamoeba coli*. Iron hematoxylin stain.

Figure 7. This immature cyst of *Entamoeba histolytica* exhibits one small resting nucleus and one larger active nucleus that appears ready to divide. A large glycogen vacuole is present. Trichrome stain.

Figure 8. *Entamoeba histolytica* (large race). The mature cyst shown in this photomicrograph contains four resting nuclei, only one of which is visible at this focal level. The finely granular cytoplasm and the smooth, almost round chromatoidal body are typical for this species. Iron hematoxylin stain.

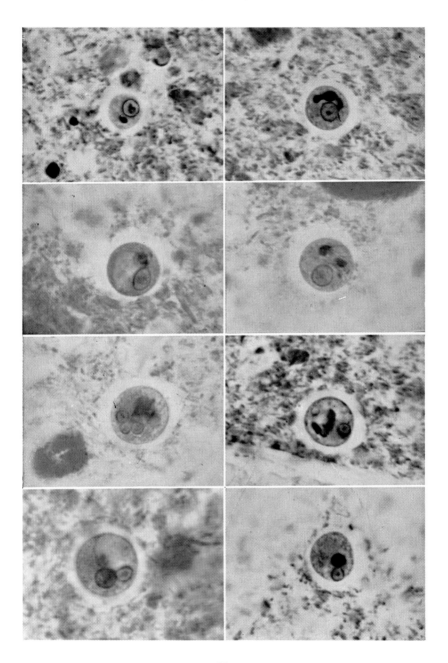

Color Plate VIII

Figure 1. *Entamoeba coli* (trophozoite). The nuclear chromatin is very course and is irregularly distributed. The nuclear karyosome is eccentric in position. A short, blunt pseudopod appears adjacent to the nucleus. Iron hematoxylin stain.

Figure 2. *Entamoeba coli* (trophozoite). The nuclear karyosome demonstrates heavy deposits of chromatin in a rather diffuse pattern. The vacuolated cytoplasm is usual in the trophozoites of this species. Iron hematoxylin stain.

Figure 3. This large trophozoite of *Entamoeba coli* shows remarkably even distribution of the cytoplasmic granules and a nucleus with a dense, compact karyosome, which is only slightly eccentric in position. Note again the absence of any ingested red blood cells. Iron hematoxylin stain.

Figure 4. *Entamoeba coli* (trophozoite). The heavy deposits of chromatin on the inner surface of the nuclear membrane and the coarse, markedly eccentric karyosome are characteristic of the motile forms of this species. Compare with the nuclear structure of the trophozoites of *Entamoeba histolytica* shown on Color Plates I and II. Iron hematoxylin stain.

Figure 5. Compare this large trophozoite of *Entamoeba coli* with the considerably smaller one shown in Figure 1. Also compare the sizes and various morphologic features of the trophozoites of *E. coli*, shown on this Color ' Plate, with those of *Entamoeba histolytica*, shown on Color Plates I, and II. Iron hematoxylin stain.

Figure 6. The trophozoite of *Entamoeba coli* was grown from culture. The karyosomal chromatin is entirely dispersed, and deposits of chromatin lining the nuclear membrane are heavy. The cytoplasmic granules are less coarse than is usual in trophozoites of this species found on direct stool examination. Iron hematoxylin stain.

Figure 7. *Entamoeba coli* (trophozoite). The nuclear structure with coarse chromatin material and a very eccentrically placed karyosome is typical, as is the presence of large food vacuoles and ingested bacteria in the cytoplasm. Iron hematoxylin stain.

Figure 8. *Entamoeba coli* (trophozoite). The sluggish motility that characterizes trophozoites of this species is suggested by the rather blunt pseudopod seen here. The other morphologic features of the trophozoite shown in this photomicrograph are equally characteristic. Iron hematoxylin stain.

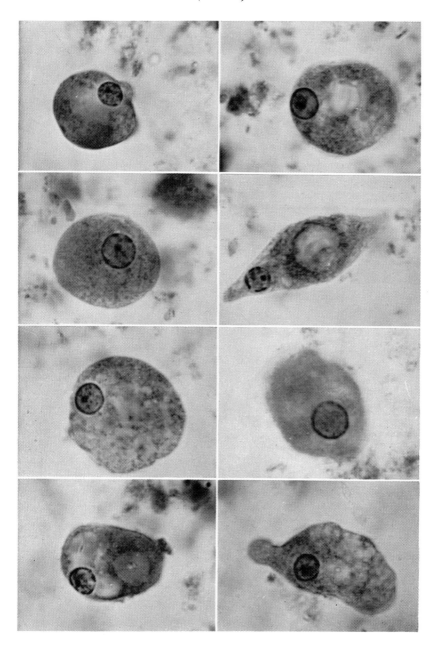

Color Plate IX

Figure 1. This large semimature cyst of *Entamoeba coli* exhibits the coarse, but evenly distributed, cytoplasmic granules so characteristic of the more mature cysts of this species. Compare with the spongy alveolar cytoplasm seen in the cysts of *Entamoeba histolytica*. Four of the seven nuclei present are visible in this focal plane. Iron hematoxylin stain.

Figure 2. Contrast the cytoplasmic structure of this very young, binucleate cyst of *Entamoeba coli* with that of the much larger and more mature cyst shown in Figure 1. Notice also extremely diffuse arrangement of karyosomal chromatin in the actively dividing nuclei. Iron hematoxylin stain.

Figure 3. *Entamoeba coli* (cyst). Notice the pronounced size variation between this unusually small cyst and the very large one shown in Figure 1. Two nuclei and a typically irregular chromatoidal body are seen in this plane of focus. Four additional nuclei are present in other focal planes. Iron hematoxylin stain.

Figure 4. Only three of the eight nuclei present in this mature cyst of *Entamoeba coli* are in sharp focus at this optical level. The nuclear karyosomes show an irregular arrangement of minute chromatin granules often seen in cysts of *E. coli*. A small, rather smooth chromatoidal is present. Iron hematoxylin stain.

Figure 5. Three of the eight nuclei present in this unstained cyst of *Entamoeba coli* can be distinguished in this photomicrograph. However, only two of the nuclei are in sharp focus at this optical level. Nuclei are not always so clearly seen in fresh, unstained preparations. Notice the highly refractile cyst wall.

Figure 6. Three of the eight nuclei present are clearly seen in this focal plane, and two others are faintly discernible in this iodine-stained cyst of *Entamoeba coli*. Notice that the punctate nuclear karyosomes are not all eccentric in position. An interesting size comparison is provided by the adjacent cyst of *Endolimax nana*.

Figure 7. *Entamoeba coli* (cyst). Five nuclei in focus at this optical level are grouped around a sixth, which is faintly seen in the center. Notice that the nuclear karyosomes seen here present a rather diffuse arrangement of chromatin particles. Iodine stain.

Figure 8. Five of the eight nuclei present in this mature, iodine-stained cyst of *Entamoeba coli* are clearly seen in this photomicrograph. Notice that not all of the punctate nuclear karyosomes are eccentric in position. The cyst wall is highly refractile.

72

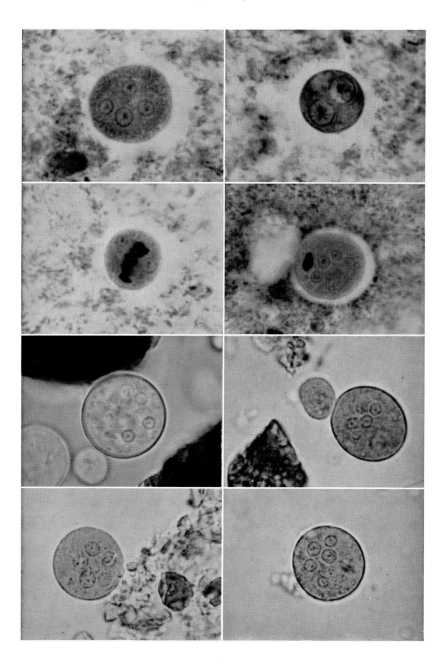

Color Plate X

Figure 1(a). *Entamoeba coli*. In this focal plane four mature resting nuclei are seen. Notice the relatively even distribution of the coarse cytoplasmic granules. Iron hematoxylin stain.

Figure 1(b). The same cyst is shown here in a slightly lower focal plane. Three additional nuclei are demonstrated, one of which is elongate and ovoid and possesses the diffuse karyosomal structure of an actively dividing nucleus. When this division is completed, the cyst will contain its full complement of eight nuclei.

Figure 2. This immature cyst of *Entamoeba coli* contains a single active nucleus and a large, irregular vacuole occupying most of the cyst. It is often impossible to distinguish such very young cysts from those of *E. histolytica*, and the differential diagnosis must be made from more mature cysts present on the same slide. Iron hematoxylin stain.

Figure 3. *Entamoeba coli* (cyst). The evenly distributed, coarse cytoplasmic granules are typical. Several small, darkly stained, irregularly shaped chromatoidals are present. Two nuclei are in sharp focus, each having an eccentric nuclear karyosome composed of small chromatin granules. Three additional nuclei are faintly visible. Iron hematoxylin stain.

Figure 4. Contrast this very large cyst of *Entamoeba coli* with the much smaller ones shown in Figures 2, 3, and 7 of Color Plate X. Several nuclei are seen in sharp or partial focus at this optical level. One nucleus is larger than the rest and shows evidence of karyokinetic activity. Iron hematoxylin stain.

Figure 5. *Entamoeba coli* (cyst). The two nuclei seen at this level of focus demonstrate typical karyosomal structure and quite delicate chromatin deposits within the nuclear membrane. The coarseness of the nuclear chromatin *in mature cysts of E. coli* has been overemphasized. Iron hematoxylin stain.

Figure 6. The diffusely vacuolated cytoplasmic structure of this possible degenerating cyst of *Entamoeba coli* is a variation not frequently seen. The cytoplasmic granules appear clumped and unusually coarse. Two resting nuclei are seen near the center of the cyst. Iron hematoxylin stain.

Figure 7. This cyst of *Entamoeba coli* contains several irregular chromatoidal bodies which demonstrate the sharp, pointed, and "splintered" ends that are quite often seen in this species but are not found in cysts of *Entamoeba histolytica*. Iron hematoxylin stain.

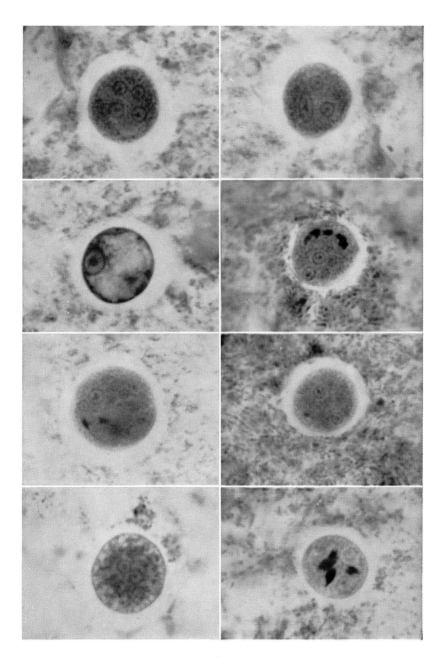

Color Plate XI

Figure l(a). The structure of this mature cyst of *Entamoeba coli* is demonstrated in this and the following two figures by serial photomicrographs made at successively lower focal levels. Two of the eight nuclei present are seen clearly in this uppermost focal plane. Iron hematoxylin stain.

Figure l(b). In this photomicrograph, made in a lower focal plane, two additional nuclei have been brought into sharp focus. Notice how serial photographic studies demonstrate and emphasize the true spherical form of amebic cysts.

Figure l(c). At this lowest optical level, a fifth nucleus is demonstrated, near the center of the cyst and partly obscured by the now imperfectly focused group of chromatoidal bodies. Note the hourglass-shaped vacuole.

Figure 2. Three resting nuclei can be seen in this cyst of *Entamoeba coli*, together with several small chromatoidal bodies. Iron hematoxylin stain.

Figure 3(a). Another mature cyst of *Entamoeba coli* is demonstrated in its entirety, in this and the following three figures, by a series of photomicrographs made in successively lower focal planes. At this uppermost optical level, two nuclei are visible. Trichrome stain.

Figure 3(b). In this photomicrograph, made in the second focal plane, two additional mature resting nuclei are in sharp focus. Notice the typical nuclear structure and arrangement of karyosomal chromatin. The dark mass at the right of the nuclei is a large, rather irregular chromatoidal body.

Figure 3(c). The fifth nucleus of the cyst is brought into view at this still deeper optical level, and the large chromatoidal body with irregular margains is now in sharp focus.

Figure 3(d). Three additional typical resting nuclei are shown in this lowest focal plane, bringing the total number to eight, the full nuclear complement of the cysts of *E. coli*.

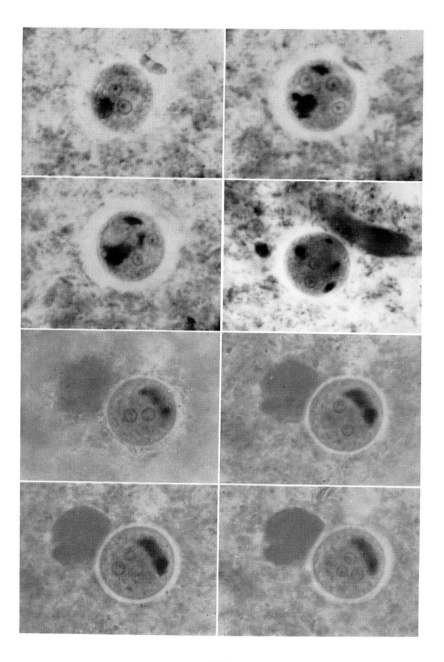

Color Plate XII

Figure 1. This immature cyst of *Entamoeba coli* exhibits a single active nucleus with coarse karyosomal chromatin, seen obliquely at the top of the cyst. A second nucleus at the opposite pole is invisible in this focal plane. Nearly the entire cyst is occupied by a huge vacuole, with many small chromatoidals lining the periphery. Iron hematoxylin stain.

Figure 2. This young cyst of *Entamoeba coli* is morphologically similar to the one shown in Figure 1, except that here both nuclei lie in the focal plane in which this photomicrograph was made. Such immature forms are not uncommon but may be very confusing to the inexperienced examiner. Iron hematoxylin stain.

Figure 3. *Entamoeba polecki* (trophozoite). The cytoplasm is coarsely vacuolated and contains ingested bacteria and other debris. Chromatin lining the nuclear membrane is moderately coarse and irregularly distributed. The nuclear karyosome is small and punctate and is central in position. Iron hematoxylin stain.

Figure 4. Karyosomal chromatin is diffusely arranged in the nucleus of this trophozoite of *Entamoeba polecki*. Notice that it is much smaller than the one shown in Figure 3. Trophozoites of this species are not distinguishable from those of *Entamoeba coli*. Iron hematoxylin stain.

Figure 5. *Entamoeba polecki* (cyst). Only one nucleus is present, as is virtually always the case in the cysts of this species. The karyosomal chromatin is densely clumped and is centrally located. The distinctive inclusion mass is seen at the left of the nucleus. Iron hematoxylin stain.

Figure 6. This small cyst of *Entamoeba polecki* contains the usual single nucleus. Heavy but evenly distributed chromatin lines the nuclear membrane. The compact karyosome is central in position. The centrally located, dark-staining inclusion mass is roughly spherical. Small chromatoidals are abundant, and some have pointed ends. Iron hematoxylin stain.

Figure 7. *Entamoeba polecki* (cyst). The chromatin lining the nuclear membrane is arranged in unusually delicate beads. The karyosome is eccentric in position, and karyosomal chromatin is dispersed. The heavy, rod-shaped chromatoidal bodies have rounded ends. A small inclusion mass lies at the left of the nucleus. Iron hematoxylin stain.

Figure 8. *Entamoeba polecki* (cyst). The nuclear chromatin is arranged in uneven plaques. The roughly spherical, dark-staining inclusion mass is clearly seen below the nucleus. The inclusion mass seen in this species is unique, not being found in the other amebae. Its nature is unknown, but it is believed not to be glycogen. Iron hematoxylin stain.

(X1320)

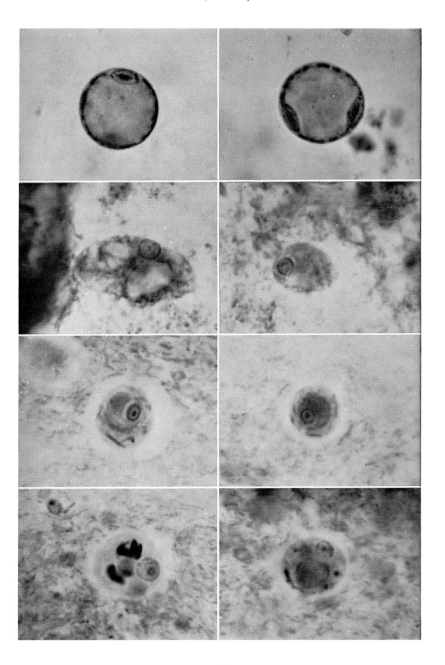

79

Color Plate XIII

Figure 1. This large trophozoite of *Iodamoeba bütschlii* exhibits a voluminous karyosome, which is eccentric in position and is actually in contact with the nuclear membrane. The cytoplasm is diffusely vacuolated and contains a variety of ingested bacteria and food debris. Iron hematoxylin stain.

Figure 3. The nucleus of this trophozoite of *Iodamoeba bütschlii* exhibits a large, smooth, slightly eccentric karyosome. Several tiny chromatin granules are faintly discernible between the karyosome and the indistinct nuclear membrane. Compare this very small trophozoite of *I. bütschlii* with the large ones shown in Figure 1 and 2. Iron hematoxylin stain.

Figure 5. A ring of tiny chromatin granules closely surrounding the nuclear karyosome of this trophozoite of *Iodamoeba bütschlii* is faintly discernible in this photomicrograph. The karyosome lies in a slightly higher focal plane than does the ring of minute chromatin granules and is therefore indistinctly focused here. Iron hematoxylin stain.

Figure 7. The nucleus of this cyst of *Iodamoeba bütschlii* is superimposed upon the glycogen vacuole. Nuclear structure is typical, with a crescent of fine chromatin granules adjacent to the slightly irregular and eccentrically placed karyosome. Iron hematoxylin stain.

Figure 2. *Iodamoeba bütschlii* (trophozoite). The large irregular karyosome is again slightly eccentric in position. The delicate nuclear membrane is unstained and invisible, causing the karyosome to appear suspended in a vacuole. The cytoplasmic structure is quite typical for this species. Iron hematoxylin stain.

Figure 4. This trophozoite of *Iodamoeba bütschlii* is of average size and again shows the characteristically vacuolated cytoplasm containing many ingested bacteria but no red blood cells. The large central karyosome is surrounded by a ring of fine chromatin granules, closely applied to the karyosome and indistinctly seen. Iron hematoxylin stain.

Figure 6. *Iodamoeba bütschlii* (cyst). The glycogen vacuole, represented by the clear space, is well shown here. It is never absent in cysts of this species. The large karyosome is central in position, and interposed between it and the invisible nuclear membrane is the usual crescentic aggregate of chromatin granules. Iron hematoxylin stain.

Figure 8. The ovoidal shape of this cyst of *Iodamoeba bütschlii* is more commonly seen than is the nearly spherical shape of the cysts shown in Figures 6 and 7. The nuclear morphology here is diagnostic, demonstrating again a crescent-shaped group of chromatin granules adjacent to the large, smooth karyosome. Iron hematoxylin stain.

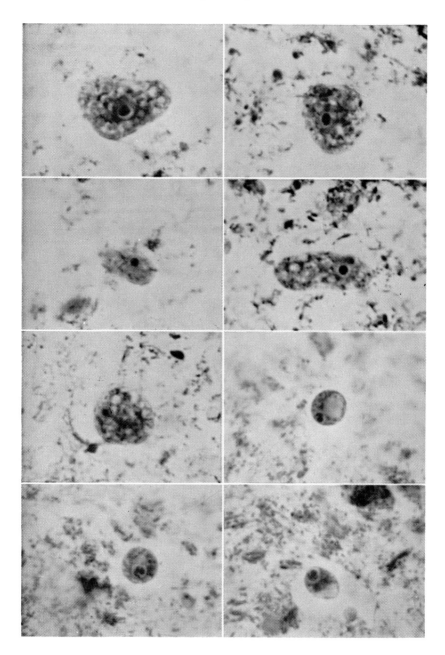

Color Plate XIV

Figure 1. The nucleus of this cyst of *Iodamoeba bütschlii* exhibits a smoothly rounded, eccentrically placed karyosome and an adjacent group of chromatin granules (above), which is roughly triangular in shape. As is often the case, individual chromatin granules are not discernible, and the group appears as a conglomerate. Iron hematoxylin stain.

Figure 3. The nucleus of this cyst of *Iodamoeba bütschlii* possess a small, ovoid karyosome, lying in an eccentric position near the inferior margin of the nucleus, adjacent to the delicate nuclear membrane. Above it are several dense chromatin granules, arranged in an irregular clump. Iron hematoxylin stain.

Figure 5. The nucleus of this cyst of *Iodamoeba bütschlii* exhibits a voluminous, perfectly round and centrally placed karyosome lacking a layer or crescent of surrounding chromatin granules. The nuclear membrane is devoid of peripheral chromatin and remains invisible. Iron hematoxylin stain.

Figure 7. *Iodamoeba bütschlii* (cyst). The nucleus is faintly distinguishable at the left side of the cyst, but nuclear detail is not visible. The unmistakable glycogen vacuole is again the clue to the identity of this iodine-stained cyst.

Figure 2. This confusing phagocyte was obtained from the stool of a patient with a rectal abscess. Notice the superficial morphologic resemblance to a large cyst of *Iodamoeba bütschlii*. The examiner will not be led into error by such pseudoparasites if careful attention is paid to the details of nuclear structure. Iron hematoxylin stain.

Figure 4. *Iodamoeba bütschlii* (cyst). The usual nuclear structure is again present, but the crescent of chromatin granules (above, right) is placed somewhat farther from the nuclear karyosome than is usual in cysts of this species. Iron hematoxylin stain.

Figure 6. The iodine-stained cyst of *Iodamoeba bütschlii* shown in this photomicrograph presents the usual ovoidal shape and conspicuous deep red-brown glycogen vacuole, which render identification certain in spite of the fact that the nucleus is not visible.

Figure 8. *Iodamoeba bütschlii* (cyst). The deep red-brown color of the glycogen vacuole seen here is obtained only when fresh material is stained with iodine. Feces preserved in formalin or concentrated by various methods usually fails to stain so deeply, and the glycogen vacuole of the cysts of *Iodamoeba* apt to be a pale yellow color.

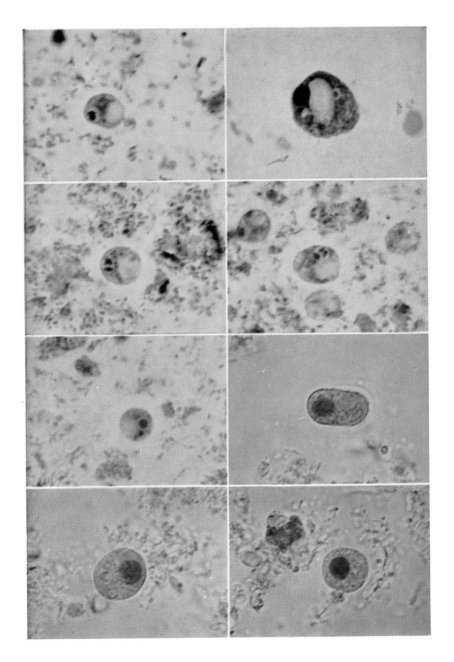

Color Plate XV

Figure 1. *Endolimax nana* (trophozoite). The nuclear karyosome is very large, irregularly shaped, and central in position. The condensation of chromatin material that nearly surrounds the nucleus is an artifact and does not represent peripheral chromatin lining the nuclear membrane. Iron hematoxylin stain.

Figure 2. *Endolimax nana* (trophozoite). Only a very narrow clear space separates the large, irregular, centrally placed karyosome from the invisible nuclear membrane. Cytoplasmic vacuoles and ingested bacteria are absent, in contrast to the usual trophozoite of this species. Iron hematoxylin stain.

Figure 3. The karyosome of this trophozoite of *Endolimax nana* is slightly irregular in shape and perhaps slightly eccentric in position, though less so than is often seen. The nuclear membrane is devoid of peripheral chromatin and remains invisible, as is usual in this species. Iron hematoxylin stain.

Figure 4. This trophozoite of *Endolimax nana* exhibits a central, round karyosome and the usual lack of chromatin lining the nuclear membrane. The cytoplasm is replaced by large vacuoles. Comparison with the cyst of *Iodamoeba bütschlii* shown in Figure 5, Plate XIV, will show that the two forms may be indistinguishable. Iron hematoxylin stain.

Figure 5. *Endolimax nana* (cyst). Three of the four nuclei present are in sharp focus in this optical plane. The large, nearly round karyosomes are characteristically eccentric in position. Intranuclear chromatin particles are not present, and the delicate nuclear membrane is invisible. Iron hematoxylin stain.

Figure 6. Two typical nuclei are seen in this cyst of *Endolimax nana*. Note the clear space that surrounds the cyst, representing the refractile cyst wall seen in fresh (unstained) and iodine-stained preparations of all the various protozoan cysts. It is never seen in the case of protozoan trophozoites. Iron hematoxylin stain.

Figure 7. Two iodine-stained cysts of *Endolimax nana* are seen in this photomicrograph. Two nuclei can be distinguished in one cyst, and only one in the other. Details of nuclear morphology are not seen. Notice the refractile cyst walls.

Figure 8. Three nuclei can be recognized in this cyst of *Endolimax nana*, but as is usual in unstained and iodine-stained preparations, nuclear detail is invisible. Such morphologic details can be seen only in preparations stained with iron hematoxylin or one of the other permanent stains.

84

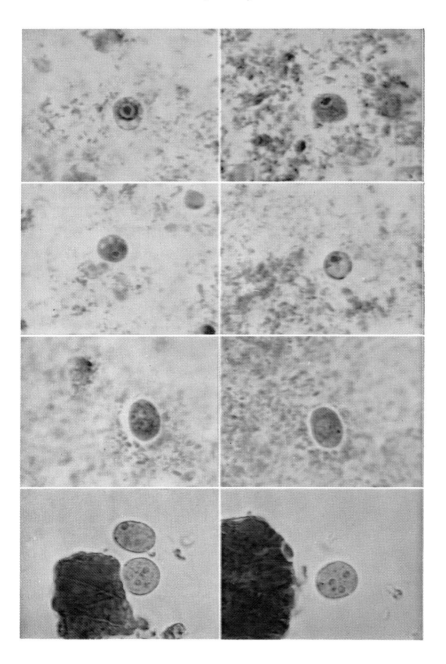

Color Plate XVI

Figure 1. *Dientamoeba fragilis* (trophozoite). The karyosomes of the two nuclei show the usual symmetrical arrangement of chromatin granules. The nuclear membranes are delicate and lack peripheral chromatin. The characteristic binucleate structure serves to distinguish this species from all other amebic trophozoites. Iron hematoxylin stain.

Figure 2. As shown in this photomicrograph, trophozoites of *Dientamoeba fragilis* are occasionally uninucleate. The nucleus seen here contains four rather irregular chromatin particles in symmetrical tetrad arrangement. As usual in this species, the cytoplasm is heavily vacuolated. Iron hematoxylin stain.

Figure 3. This trophozoite of *Dientamoeba fragilis* exhibits two small nuclei with a symmetrical tetrad arrangement of the four chromatin granules present in each. Notice that the nuclei are much smaller than in the case of the uninucleate trophozoite shown in Figure 2. Iron hematoxylin stain.

Figure 4. Here is another uninucleate trophozoite of *Dietamoeba fragilis*. The karyosome is composed of four chromatin granules, which in this instance are not uniform in size and are not entirely symmetrical in arrangement. A cyst stage of this species is not known. Iron hematoxylin stain.

Figure 5. This large trophozoite of *Dientamoeba fragilis* is binucleate, as are more than 70 percent of the trophozoites of this species. The chromatin granules of the karyosomes are irregular, compact, and asymmetrically arranged. Iron hematoxylin stain.

Figure 6. *Dientamoeba fragilis* (trophozoite). The two nuclei present exhibit karyosomes whose chromatin particles are arranged in an irregular rosette. Notice the heavily vacuolated structure of the cytoplasm. Iron hematoxylin stain.

Figure 7. The chromatin particles that comprise the karyosome in this uninucleate trophozoite of *Dientamoeba fragilis* are arranged as a narrow band across the nucleus. Iron hematoxylin stain.

Figure 8. Two nuclei are present in this trophozoite of *Dientamoeba fragilis,* but only one is sharply focused in this photomicrograph. The chromatin particles of the karyosome exhibit a rosette arrangement that is quite symmetrical. Iron hematoxylin stain.

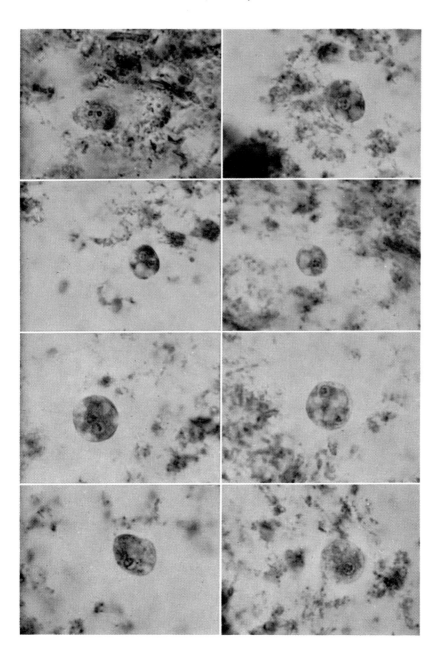

Color Plate XVII

Figure 1. *Giardia lamblia* (trophozoite). The pear-shaped body with sharply attentuated posterior end, the two large subspherical nuclei, and the short, thick median bodies lying just posterior to the nuclei all serve to make recognition easy. The flagella are not visible. Iron hematoxylin stain.

Figure 3. Four nuclei are seen near one pole (left) of this cyst of *Giardia lamblia*. Notice that the small karyosomes may be either central or eccentric in position. The large clear space surrounding the organism represents the unstained cyst wall plus shrinkage due to fixation. Iron hematoxylin stain.

Figure 5. Only two of the four nuclei present in this cyst of *Girardia lamblia* are visible in this focal plane. The axonemes and the intracytoplasmic fiagellar structures are well shown in this photomicrograph. Iron hematoxylin stain.

Figure 2. *Giardia lamblia* (trophozoite). The karyosomes are nearly central in position, but one is indistinctly seen in this focal plane. The nuclear membranes are heavy but are not provided with peripheral chromatin. The intracytoplasmic portions (axonemes) of the invisible caudal flagella divide the body into halves. Iron hematoxylin stain.

Figure 4. *Giardia lamblia* (cyst). Karyosomes of the two nuclei are eccentrically placed, and their delicate nuclear membranes are devoid of peripheral chromatin. The thick, curved fragments of the ventral sucking disk are prominent near the opposite pole of the cyst. The paired longitudinal axonemes are also visible. Iron hematoxylin stain.

Figure 6. This photomicrograph demonstrates once more the diagnostic morphologic features that make *Giardia lamblia* one of the most easily recognized of the intestinal protozoan parasites. The two nuclei visible in this iron hematoxylin stained cyst have smoothly rounded karyosomes that are almost exactly central in position.

Figure 7. *Giardia lamblia* (cyst). The karsosomes of the two nuclei visible in this focal plane are central in position. These karyosomes are pink in color when viewed through the microscope in this trichrome-stained preparation, but the color is very difficult to reproduce in the photomicrographs.

Figure 8. *Giardia lamblia* (cyst). The axonemes and other intracytoplasmic structures are unusually well seen in this iodine-stained cyst, though much less detail is visible than in preparations stained with iron hematoxylin or one of the other permanent stains.

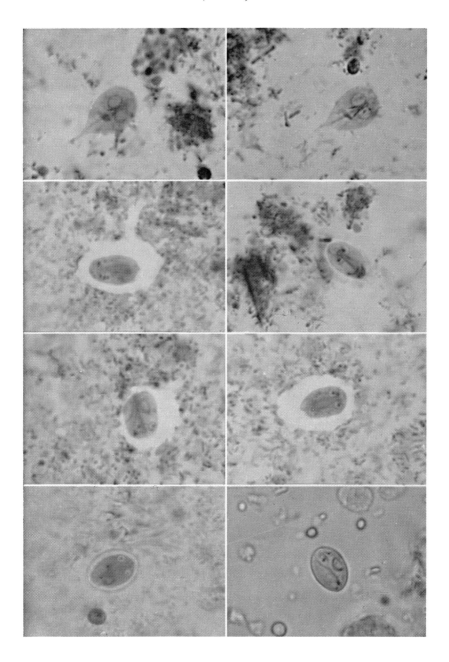

Color Plate XVIII

Figure 1. *Chilomastix mesnili* (trophozoite). The single nucleus contains a small eccentric karyosome, and some chromatin granules are present on the nuclear membrane. Cytostomal fibrils are seen below the nucleus. This trophozoite is less abruptly tapered toward the posterior end than is usual in the living organism. Iron hematoxylin stain.

Figure 2. *Chilomastix mesnili* (trophozoite). The nucleus exhibits a small, centrally placed karyosome. The flagella are not visible in this iron hematoxylin stained preparation. Notice the cytostomal fibrils and the sharply pointed posterior end.

Figure 3. *Chilomastix mesnili* (cyst). The characteristically lemon-shaped cyst contains one nucleus with a large irregularly shaped karyosome, which is eccentric in position. Notice the cytostomal fibrils. Iron hematoxylin stain.

Figure 4. This iodine-stained cyst of *Chilomastix mesnili* demonstrates clearly the characteristic pear-shaped or lemon-shaped appearance that results from the blunt prominence at one pole of the cyst. Nuclear detail is not visible, and cytostomal fibrils are not easily recognized, but the unmistakable shape renders identification easy.

Figure 5. The leucocyte shown in this photomicrograph, made from a preparation stained with iodine, is one of a great variety of cellular structures found in feces. Such cells are a trap which may snare the unwary or inexperienced examiner. The coarsely granular cytoplasm and the lack of refractile cyst wall are helpful distinguishing features.

Figure 6. The costa is well stained and easily recognized in each of these two trophozoites of *Trichomonas hominis*. The nuclear chormatin is unevenly distributed and the nuclear membranes are delicate. One or two flagella are faintly visible, but the axostyles are not well seen in this focal plane. Iron hematoxylin stain.

Figure 7. This photomicrograph, made from a fecal suspension stained with iodine, demonstrates a structure, probably a pollen grain or a diatom, occasionally encountered. Despite its regular shape and obviously organic composition, the lack of specific morphologic features should prevent such bodies from being mistaken for an intestinal parasite.

Figure 8. Another of the great variety of confusing structures seen in feces is shown here. Note the lack of a refractile cyst wall. Careful attention to size, nuclear structure, and other morphologic details, or the lack of them, will prevent mistaking such objects for a parasite, even though specific identification may not be possible. Iodine stain.

90

(X1320)

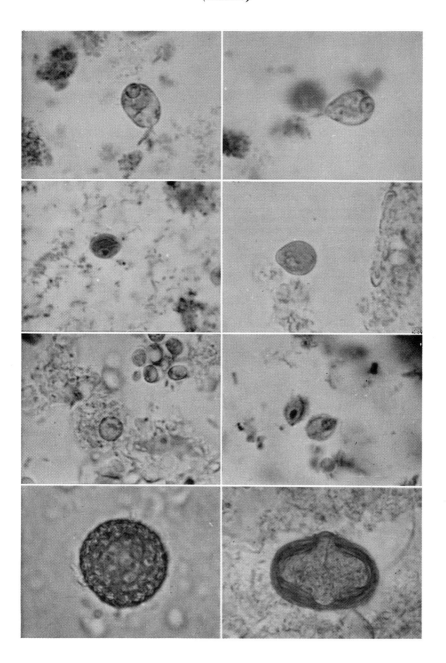

Color Plate XIX

Figure 1. *Blastocystis hominis*. This organism, possibly a protozoan, is a common commensal in the digestive tract of man. It may be confused with an encysted protozoan parasite if the examiner is inexperienced. The structureless central portion resembles a vacuole appearing to contain homogeneous material. Iron hematoxylin stain.

Figure 2. As shown in this photomicrograph, *Blastocystis hominis* may vary greatly in size, shape, and other morphologic details. A wide variety of other tiny yeast forms are commonly found in feces but are unlikely to cause confusion in view of their very small size. Iron hematoxylin stain.

Figure 3. *Blastocystis hominis* from a preparation stained with iodine is demonstrated here. The larger of the two blastocysts exhibits several distinct nuclei arranged at the periphery, whereas the smaller one contains only one nucleus.

Figure 4. This cellular pseudoparasite was obtained from the stool of a patient with idiopathic ulcerative colitis. To avoid the error of identifying such structures as a protozoan parasite, one must search for and recognize the specific morphologic features and nuclear details of the various species and forms. Iron hematoxylin stain.

Figure 5. This photomicrograph demonstrates a common polymorphonuclear leucocyte, from a fecal suspension stained with iodine. Compare with the similar cells appearing in Figure 1 of Plate I. Such cells are often confused with an amebic cyst.

Figure 6. This oocyst of *Isospora belli* is the immature form usually found in freshly passed feces. The ellipsoidal oocyst contains only an unsegmented mass of granular protoplasm in this unstained preparation.

Figure 7. Here is another immature oocyst of *Isospora belli*. This species is often mistakenly identified as *Isospora hominis*. As shown in this photomicrograph, *Isospora belli* stains slowly and unevenly with iodine if the oocyst wall is intact.

Figure 8. This mature, unstained oocyst of *Isospora belli* contains two sporocysts, each of which in turn contains four sporocysts of *I. hominis* have almost escaped the oocyst by the time they appear in the feces, where they are seen singly, or in pairs, devoid of an oocyst wall.

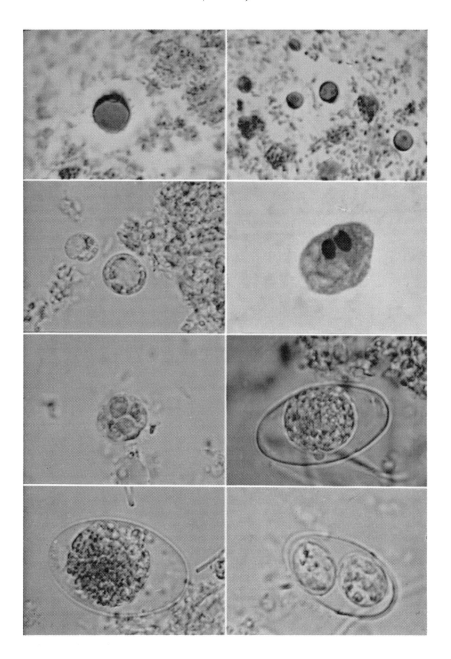

Color Plate XX

Figure 1. *Eimeria stiedae.* The iodine-stained oocyst shown here contains only the unsegmented sporoblast. *Because of its large size, it was necessary to photograph this protozoan species at the lower magnification used for the helminth ova.* This species of Coccidia is closely related to *Isospora belli* and *Isospora hominis.*

Figure 2. This nearly mature iodine-stained oocyst of *Eimeria stiedae* contains four sporocysts, in contrast to the two contained in the mature oocyst of *Isospora*. Each sporocyst of *E. stiedae* contains only two sporozoites, instead of the four found in each sporocyst of *Isospora*. A prominent micropyle is seen at the narrow end of the oocyst.

Figure 3. The structure shown in this photomicrograph is quite commonly encountered in the feces. It is probably a pollen grain. It is unlikely that such a curious, spiny object could be mistaken for a parasite form. Iodine stain.

Figure 4. The cilia, the cytostome, the elongate macronucleus, and the large food vacuole are all discernible in this iodine-stained trophozoite of *Balantiadium coli*. *Because of its large size, it is necessary to show this protozoan at the lower magnification otherwise reserved for the helminth ova.*

Figure 5. The ellipsoidal macronucleus and the large food vacuole are readily distinguished in this iodine-stained cyst of *Balantidium coli.* Cilia are not visible here but may be seen in newly encysted organisms.

Figure 6. The ellipsoidal macronucleus appears quite round in this small iodine-stained cyst of *Balantidium coli* because it is viewed in cross section. The cysts of this species vary considerably in size and may appear to be spherical as shown here, or ellipsoidal, as in Figure 5.

Figure 7. *Balantidium coli* (trophozoite). The prominent cytostome, the cilia, and the macronucleus are well demonstrated in this unstained trophozoite. The macronucleus appears nearly spherical, as it is seen in cross section. This species is the largest protozoan form parasitizing man.

Figure 8. This iron hematoxylin stained trophozoite of *Balantidium coli* demonstrates the ususal morphologic features. *B. coli* is the only member of the Class Ciliatea to parasitize man. It is sometimes confused with smaller coprozoic ciliates, which may contaminate water in which feces have been collected or water is used in preparing fecal films.

94

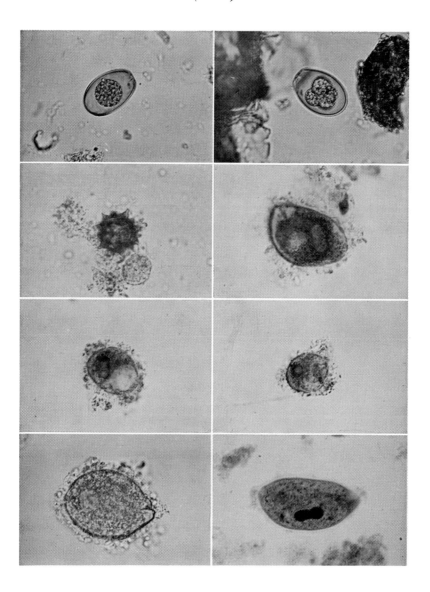

Color Plate XXI

Figure 1. This photomicrograph demonstrates an unsegmented, unstained egg of *Enterobius vermicularis*. The eggs of this species are elongate, ovoidal, and somewhat flattened on the ventral side.

Figure 2. This fully embryonated egg of *Enterobius vermicularis* has been stained with iodine, which readily penetrates the eggshell and kills the contained larva. Formalin solutions in common use do not penetrate the eggshell or kill the embryo, which may proceed to development of an actively motile larva while kept in such solutions.

Figure 3. *Enterobius vermicularis*. The larva of this fully embryonated, iodine-stained egg appears to be emerging from the eggshell, but this is an artifact resulting from pressure on the coverslip.

Figure 4. *Enterobius vermicularis*. Again the larva has been made to appear as though it were "hatching" by tapping sharply on the coverslip, thus forcing the larva partly through the fragil shell. Iodine stain.

Figure 5(a). Two unstained eggs of *Enterobius vermicularis* are seen here floating so that they are viewed "on end." This and the following photomicrograph are shown to demonstrate the confusing appearance that may result when any of the helminth eggs are seen "on end" or from an unusual angle.

Figure 5(b). The same two eggs of *Enterobius vermicularis* are shown here after gently tapping the coverslip so as to cause them to float into the more usual horizontal position.

Figure 6. This is an unfertilized, unstained egg of *Ascaris lumbricoides*. The golden brown color results from bile staining. Internally the egg is made up of refractile, disorganized granules of variable size.

Figure 7. The fertilized, iodine-stained egg of *Ascaris lumbricoides* shown in this photomicrograph has progressed to the two-cell stage. Notice the coarsely mammillated external layer.

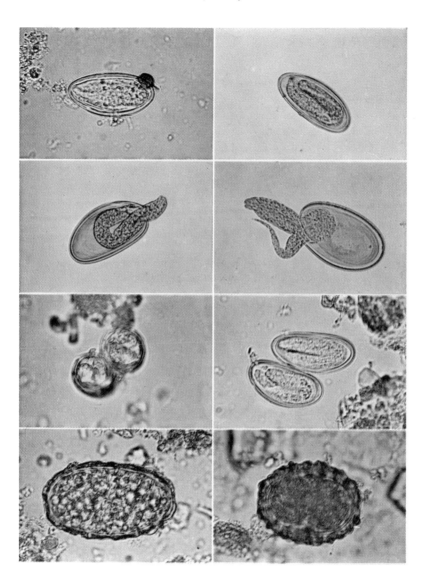

Color Plate XXII

Figure 1. *Ascaris lumbricoides.* The albuminoid external layer of this unfertilized, iodine-stained egg is even more coarsely mammillated than usual. Infertile eggs of *Ascaris* may present a bizarre appearance which makes them easily confused with various plant structures and pseudoparasites found in feces.

Figure 2. Here is another infertile, iodine-stained egg of *Ascaris lumbricoides.* The unfertilized eggs of this species are quite fragile and may be broken, or the mamillated external layer may be removed by pressure on the coverslip. In some cases the albuminoid external shell is never added.

Figure 3. This unstained, fertilized, unsegmented egg of *Ascaris lumbricoides* lacks its mammillated external layer, and is spoken of as being decorticated. Such eggs resemble those of *Necator americanus* (hookworm), but the remaining inner shell is always much thicker than the shell of a hookworm egg.

Figure 4. The mammillated external shell is still present in this fertilized, unstained egg of *Ascaris lumbricoides.* Segmentation has progressed to the four-cell stage. Like the egg shown in Figure 3, this egg lacks the usual degree of bile staining and appears nearly colorless.

Figure 5. This decorticated egg of *Ascaris lumbricoides* is fertilized but unsegmented, and it is stained with iodine. Notice that the space between the external shell and the developing embryo stains readily with iodine. This is in contrast to the eggs of *Necator americanus* and may serve to help distinguish the two species.

Figure 6. *Ascaris lumbricoides.* This fertilized, unsegmented egg has retained the mammillated external layer. This is perhaps the most common and typical form in which the eggs of *Ascaris* are seen. Iodine stain.

Figure 7. Division of the embryo has progressed to the four-cell stage in this iodine-stained egg of *Ascaris lumbricoides.* The irregular external albuminoid layer is intact.

Figure 8. The partly decorticated egg of *Ascaris* shown here contains a fully developed first-stage larva. Such larvae survive and remain motile in strong solutions of formalin for long periods, provided the eggshell remains intact. Iodine, however, readily penetrates the egg and kills the larva.

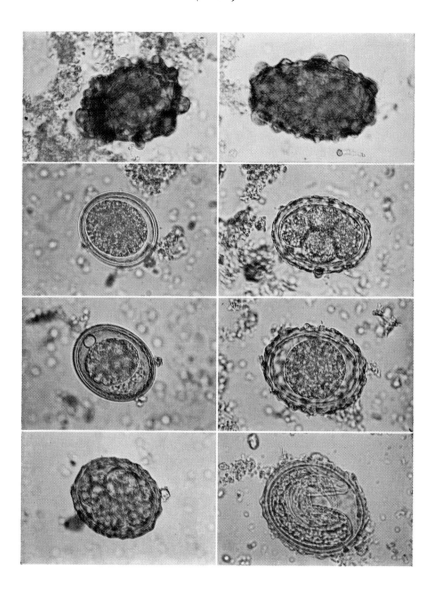

Color Plate XXIII

Figure 1. *Necator americanus* (hookworm). This iodine-stained egg demonstrates clearly that in this species the space between the thin outer shell and the developing embryo is not stained by iodine. Contrast with the iodine-stained eggs of *Ascaris lumbricoides* shown in Figures 5, 6, 7, and 8 of Color Plate XXII.

Figure 2. *Necator americanus.* As shown in this photomicrograph, unstained hookworm eggs are quite colorless, not being stained by the bile pigments present in the feces. Freshly passed eggs are usually unsegmented, as in this example, or they may have reached an early segmentation stage.

Figure 3. *Trichostrongylus orientalis.* As demonstrated in this photomicrograph, the eggs of this species are like those of the closely related hookworms, in that iodine does not stain the space between the external shell and the developing embryo. However, *Trichostrongylus* eggs are larger, and one end of the egg is somewhat pointed.

Figure 4. *Trichostrongylus orientalis.* Segmentation in this unstained egg has progressed to an early morula stage. Compare with the hookworm eggs shown in Figure 1 and 2 of this Plate, and Figures 1 and 2 of Color Plate XXIV, and note that eggs of *Trichostrongylus* are considerably larger, and have a tendency for one end of the egg to be pointed.

Figure 5. This iodine-stained egg of *Trichostrongylus* contains a nearly developed rhabditoid larva. The egg is somewhat broader and shorter than most eggs of this species but retains the tendency for one end to be pointed. Accurate differentiation of the several species of *Trichostrongylus* cannot be made from the eggs alone.

Figure 6. *Trichuris (Trichocephalus) trichiura.* This photomicrograph shows the characteristically barrel-shaped egg with the refractile intraluminar prominences, usually called polar plugs, at either end. These features make this one of the most easily recognized of all the helminth eggs. Iodine stain.

Figure 7. This fertilized, iodine-stained egg of *Trichuris trichiura* demonstrates clearly the triple shell and the bipolar unstained prominences having the appearance of mucoid plugs.

Figure 8. This photomicrograph of an unstained, infertile egg of *Trichuris trichiura* shows the usual brown or yellow-brown color of the eggs of this species. The color is probably due in part to bile staining.

100

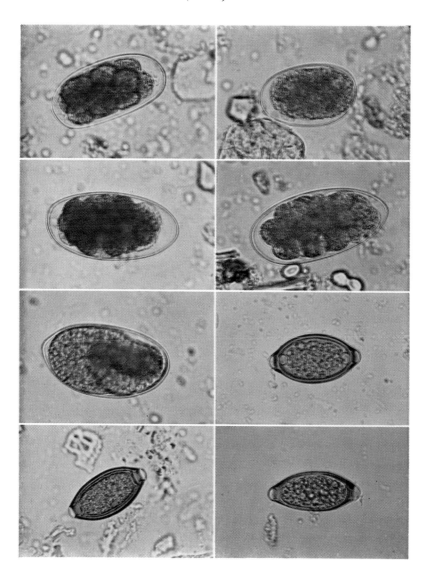

Color Plate XXIV

Figure 1. *Necator americanus.* Notice the eggshell as well as the space between the shell and the developing embryo remains entirely free of the iodine stain, whereas the embryo itself stains readily.

Figure 2. Another iodine-stained egg of *Necator americanus.* Like the hookworm egg shown in Figure 1, this photomicrograph is included here to provide easy comparison with eggs of *Strongyloides stercoralis* shown in Figures 4 and 5 of this Plate.

Figure 3. The photomicrograph shows the anterior and posterior ends of a rhabditoid larva of *Necator americanus.* Notice the long buccal chamber, which serves to distinguish the rhabditoid hookworm larvae from those of *Strongyloides stercoralis.*

Figure 4. Here is the rarely seen egg of *Strongyloides stercoralis*, containing the usual fully developed first-stage larva. The eggs, which are very similar in appearance to those of hookworm, are found in the stool only in case of severe diarrhea or after strong purgation. Note that only the developing embryo is stained by the iodine.

Figure 5. This unstained egg of *Strongyloides* demonstrates well the more rounded shape and smaller size of the eggs of this species, as compared to hookworm eggs. *Strongyloides* eggs are rarely found in the feces, since the eggs almost invariably hatch within the intestine, and only the rhabditoid, or occasionally the filariform larvae, will be seen.

Figure 6. The anterior end of this rhabditoid larva of *Strongyloides stercoralis* demonstrates clearly the short buccal chamber that distinguishes it from the rhabditoid larvae of the hookworms and *Trichostrongylus,* as well as from the free-living *Rhabditis* species. Iodine stain.

Figure 7. This iodine-stained rhabditoid larva of the free-living species, *Rhabditis hominis* exhibits a long buccal chamber like that of the rhabditoid larva of hookworm. It contrasts with the short buccal chamber of *Strongyloides* larvae. *Rhabditis* larvae of greatly varying size and stage of developement may be found in a single stool specimen.

Figure 8. This unstained rhabditoid larva of *Rhabditis hominis* is considerably larger than the one shown in Figure 7. The very long and thickly cuticularized buccal chamber is easily seen, as is the bulbar swelling in the middle of the anterior club-shaped portion of the esophagus.

102

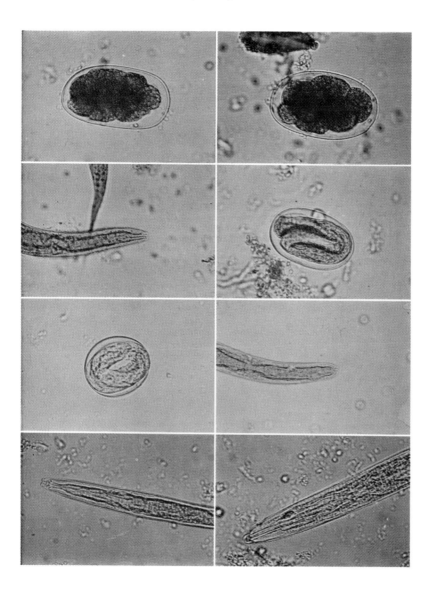

Color Plate XXV

Figure 1. This unstained egg of *Taenia saginata* exhibits the distinctive, dark brown, thick-walled, and radially striated shell. The egg is surrounded by the hyaline embryonic membrane, sometimes called a "mucous sheath." This sheath, or envelope, is not always present, but when seen it aids in the identification of the eggs of *Taenia* species.

Figure 2. The iodine-stained egg of *Taenia saginata* shown in this photomicrograph also demonstrates the hyaline mucous envelope, radially striated shell, and spherical or subspherical shape that make these eggs readily recognizable. Eggs of *Taenia saginata* cannot be distinguished from those of *Taenia solium*.

Figure 3. *Diphyllobothrium latum.* The broadly ovoidal egg with a prominent operculum and a small knob, or boss, on the abopercular end is easily recognized from this photomicrograph. The unstained egg shown here is immature and contains an undeveloped embryo.

Figure 4. This egg of *Diphyllobothrium latum* has been stained with iodine. The moderately thick shells of the eggs of this species are quite fragile and are easily broken by pressure on the coverslip. By tapping gently on the coverslip, the examiner may force open the operculum and thus render it easily visible.

Figure 5. The unstained egg of *Hymenolepis nana* shown in this photomicrograph is nearly spherical, but the eggs of this species may be subspherical or ovoidal. Several of the six hooklets present in the oncosphere can be distinguished in this focal plane.

Figure 6. *Hymenolepis nana.* The smooth, hyaline outer shell is lined by granular material and separated from the inner envelope containing the oncosphere by a rather wide clear space. Within this clear space, originating from the polar thickenings of the inner envelope, are seen the characteristic polar filaments. Iodine stain.

Figure 7. *Hymenolepis diminuta.* This unstained egg demonstrates the much larger size and complete lack of polar filaments that serve to distinguish eggs of this species from those of *H. nana.* The wide space between the transparent outer shell and the inner envelope enclosing the oncosphere is filled with a colorless gelatinous matrix.

Figure 8. *Hymenolepis diminuta.* At least four of the six hooklets present in the oncosphere are readily seen in this photomicrograph. Notice the absence of polar filaments. Small polar thickenings are present on the inner envelope but are not visible here because they are not in this optical plane. Iodine stain.

(X430)

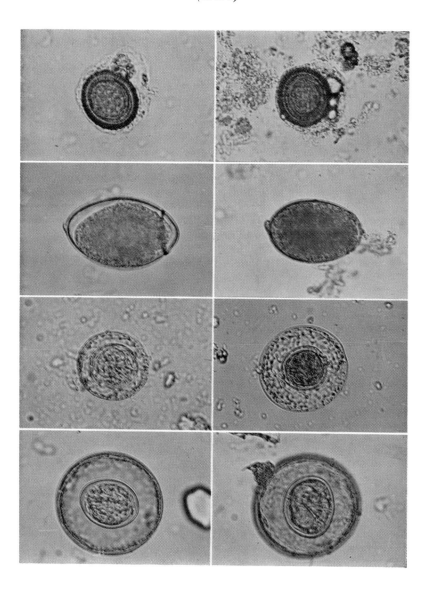

Color Plate XXVI

Figure 1. This photomicrograph shows a group of vegetable cells (string beans), a type commonly found in the feces. Their rather uniform size and distinctive structure make them easily recognizable. Iodine stain.

Figure 2. Spiral vessels ("vegetable spirals") of the spirovascular bundle of plants, such as those seen in this photomicrograph, are frequently encountered in examinations of the feces. The unstained spiral shown here is tightly coiled, but these common structures are often seen partly or completely uncoiled.

Figure 3. The unstained structure shown here is sometimes called a "stone cell" or "colloidal cell." Commonly found in the feces, its refractile quality, somewhat amorphous structure, and irregular shape should prevent its being confused with a helminth egg.

Figure 4. The "stone cell" demonstrated in this photomicrograph has been stained with iodine. Within a short time, heat from the substage lamp of the microscope may cause these bodies to swell markedly and become almost completely amorphous.

Figure 5. Plant hairs such as the one shown here are sometimes mistaken for a larval nematode. Recognition of the minute central canal extending the entire length of the structure, and the thick refractile wall, should prevent such errors. Vegetable hairs are quite pointed at one end but are blunt and irregular at the other. Iodine stain.

Figure 6. The color and conspicuous striations of the incompletely digested, unstained muscle fiber shown here are characteristic. Such muscle fibers should be recognized and, when present in the excessive numbers, should be reported, for they may indicate insufficiency of pancreatic digestion or other important disease.

Figure 7. The striations of this poorly digested muscle fiber have been rendered more distinct by the iodine stain. While it is not unusual to find small numbers of undigested or partly digested muscle fibers in normal stools, they should be reported when present in excessive numbers.

Figure 8. This unstained parenchymatous plant cell represents a type frequently found in the feces. Such vegetable cells may superficially resemble a helminth egg and may mistakenly be identified as such by a careless or inexperienced examiner. They rarely have as regular contours as the eggs of helminths.

106

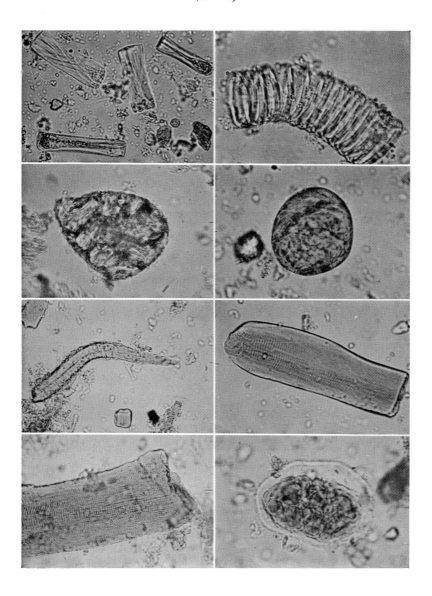

Color Plate XXVII

Figure 1. This tiny pseudoparasite, probably a diatom, possesses regular morphology and structare that identify it as an organic body. It is a structure occasionally found in the feces, and it is sometimes confused with an amebic cyst or with one of the tiny trematode eggs shown in Figure 3 through 8 of this Plate. Iodine stain.

Figure 3. The unstained egg of *Clonorchis (Opisthorchis) sinensis* shown in this photomicrograph presents the characteristic pyriform shape, the prominent operculum, and the small knob or boss at the abopercular end that serve to distinguish the eggs of this species.

Figure 5. *Heterophyes heterophyes.* As seen here, eggs of this species are slightly smaller than those of *Clonorchis* and lack the distinctive "shouldering" of that species. The tiny, ovoidal eggs of *Heterophyes* show no definite boss at the abopercular end, but a minute prominence formed by an extension of the shell may be detected. Unstained.

Figure 7. This photomicrograph demonstrates the unstained egg of *Metagonimus yokogawai*. Smallest of the important helminth eggs, this egg lacks a boss at the broad (abopercular) end and exhibits an ovoid or slightly pyriform shape. No "shouldering" is seen, and the operculum is not distinct.

Figure 2. The spores of the fungus of corn smut, shown in this photomicrograph, are another type of small body that might be mistaken for a parasite form. It is sometimes encountered in stool specimens. Unstained.

Figure 4. This iodine-stained egg of *Clonorchis sinensis* exhibits the distinctly convex operculum that fits into a rimmed extension of the shell, producing the marked "shouldering" that is a unique and distinctive morphologic feature of the eggs of this species. The boss at the abopercular end of this egg is quite small and is eccentrically placed.

Figure 6. Careful comparison of this iodine-stained egg of *Heterophyes heterophyes* with the eggs of *Clonorchis sinensis* (Figs. 3 and 4) and with the eggs of *Metagonimus yokogawai* (Figs. 7 and 8) will reveal minor morphologic differences that assist in distinguishing these tiny trematode eggs, which so closely resemble one another.

Figure 8. In order to facilitate further comparison of morphologic features, this single photomicrograph demonstrates together the iodine-stained eggs of *Clonochis sinensis* (left) and *Metagonimus yokogawai* (right).

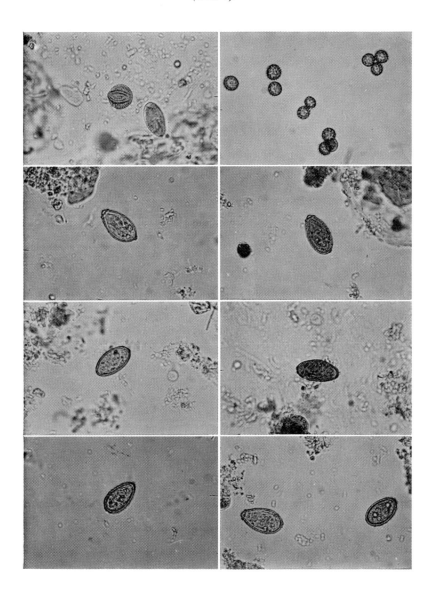

Color Plate XXVIII

Figure 1. This operculate egg, found in the stools of a soldier returning from Korea, has been identified by several experts as an echinostome egg, probably that of *Echinochasmus perfoliatus*. Echinostome eggs are not of specific diagnostic value, and positive identification is best made from the adult worms following anthelmintic therapy. Unstained.

Figure 2. The rhomboidal shape and distinct vitelline cells of this unstained, operculate egg identify it as a paramphistomid egg, probably that of *Gastrodiscoides hominis*, according to several consulting parasitologists.

Figure 3. *Paragonimus westermani*. This iodine-stained egg demonstrates the broadly ovoidal shape, with the maximum width nearer the operculum (right) than the equator of the egg and the thickening of the shell at the abopercular end, that are characteristic of the eggs of the species.

Figure 4. This unstained egg of *Paragonimus westermani* exhibits the rather small but distinct and slightly flattened operculum (left), typical shape, and thickening of the shell at the abopercular end that are the distinctive morphologic features of the eggs of this species.

Figure 5. Compare this unstained egg of *Paragonimus kellicotti* with those of *P. westermani* shown in Figures 3 and 4, and note that the egg of *P. kellicotti* is somewhat more regularly ovoidal and lacks the marked degree of thickening of the shell at the abopercular end. The partly open operculum is an artifact caused by pressure on the coverslip.

Figure 6. *Dicrocoelium dendriticum*. As demonstrated in this photomicrograph, eggs of this species are operculate, thick shelled, and deep golden brown in color. Unstained.

Figure 7. *Macracanthorhynchus hirudinaceus*. Eggs of this species are symmetrically ovoidal, thick shelled, and have three embryonic envelopes, as demonstrated in this photomicrograph. Unstained.

Figure 8. *Macracanthorhynchus hirudinaceus*. This fully embryonated egg, with enclosed acanthor, has been stained with iodine. This species, which belongs to a separate phylum (Acanthocephala), is included here with the trematodes only because technical reasons prevented placing it elsewhere in the photographic series.

110

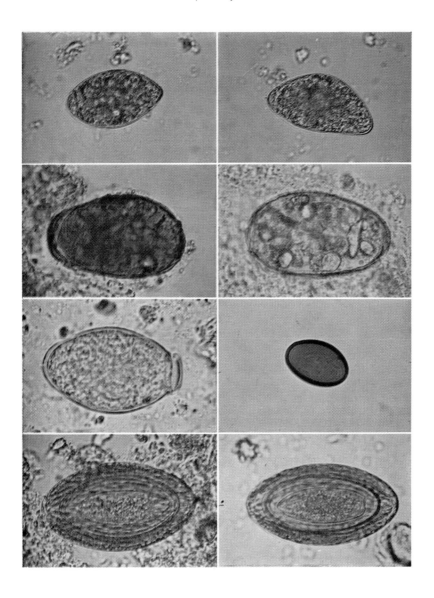

Color Plate XXIX

Figure 1. *Schistosoma mansoni.* As demonstrated in this photomicrograph, eggs of this species are elongate, ovoidal, somewhat yellowish brown bodies with a transparent shell and a characteristic thornlike lateral spine. Confusion may result when the egg is viewed in a projection that causes the distinctive lateral spine to be hidden under the body of the egg. Unstained.

Figure 2. This photomicrograph demonstrates an iodine-stained egg of *Schistosoma mansoni.* The conspicuous lateral spine and large size of the eggs of this species make it one of the most easily recognized of all the helminth eggs. At times, however, they may be confused with undigested vegetable objects.

Figure 3. This iodine-stained egg of the *Schistosoma haematobium* exhibits the broadly ovoidal shape and characteristic small terminal spine, which serve to make recognition of this species easy.

Figure 4. The unstained egg of *Schistosoma haematobium* shown in this photomicrograph is somewhat narrower and more elongate than the egg of this species demonstrated in Figure 3. Again, notice the small terminal spine at the lower pole of the egg.

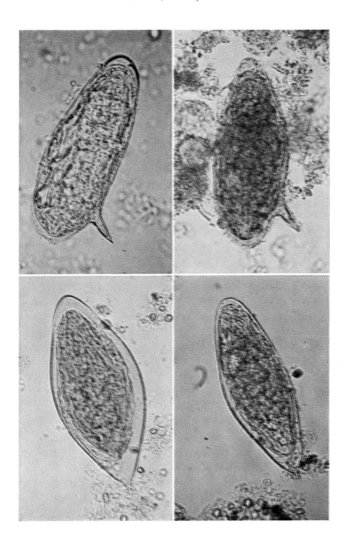

Color Plate XXX

Figure 1. In this egg of *Schistosoma mansoni* the transparent shell is easily distinguished from the enclosed miracidium. The very sharply pointed and prominent lateral spine is an unmistakable diagnostic feature. Iodine stain.

Figure 2. *Schistosoma japonicum.* As demonstrated here, the eggs of this species are distinctly ovoidal in shape and are somewhat smaller than those of the other schistosomes. Eggs of *S. japonicum* are usually described as having an abbreviated lateral spine, but it is extremely difficult to see and is not visible in this photomicrograph. Note the fully developed miracidium within the shell. Unstained.

Figure 3. This photomicrograph of an iodine-stained egg of *Schistosoma japonicum* again demonstrates that the minute lateral spine is rarely seen, being visible as a tiny recurved hook only when the egg is properly oriented and is viewed in a suitable projection. Notice the secretion of internal glands sticking to the outside of the shell.

Figure 4. The very large egg of *Fasciolopisis buski* is presented in this photomicrograph. Eggs of this species are exceeded in size only by those of *Fasciola gigantica* (Plate XXXII, Figs. 1 and 2) and are only slightly larger than those of *Fasciola hepatica* (Plate XXXI, Figs. 3 and 4). The operculum (top, right) of this unstained egg has been detached.

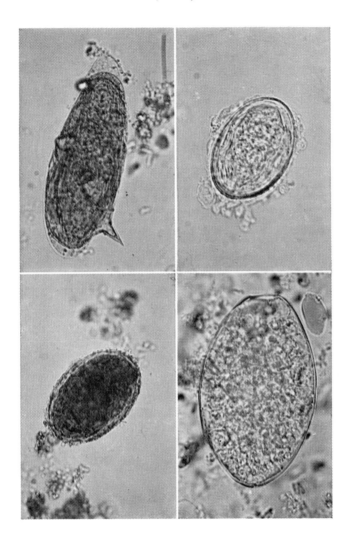

Color Plate XXXI

Figure 1. Another unstained egg of *Fasciolopis buski* is shown in this photomicrograph. The open but still attached operculum appearing at the upper pole of the egg (top) is an artifact deliberately produced by pressure on the coverslip, for the purpose of making the small operculum more easily visible.

Figure 2. The operculum of this iodine-stained egg of *Fasciolopsis buski* is intact, and can be recognized as a small crescent at the upper pole of the egg (top). The eggs of this species, as well as those of the other Fasciolidae, stain readily and deeply with iodine.

Figure 3. An unstained egg of *Fasciola hepatica* is shown here, with the tiny operculum being faintly visible at the upper pole of the egg (top). Compare the structure and arrangement of the yolk cells with those of the eggs of *Fasciolopis buski* shown in Figures 1 and 2.

Figure 4. *Fasciola hepatica*. Comparison with the eggs of *Fasciolopsis buski* shown in Figures 1 and 2 demonstrates that the eggs of this species are generally slightly smaller and somewhat more narrow. The operculum of this iodine-stained egg is located at the upper pole of the egg (top) but is recognized with difficulty.

(X430)

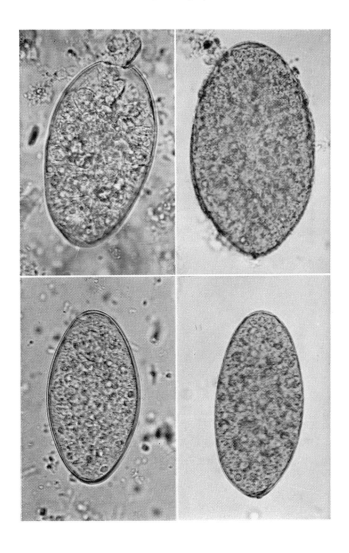

Color Plate XXXII

Figure 1. This is an unstained egg of *Fasciola gigantica*. Largest of the helminth eggs, it closely resembles those of *Fasciolopsis buski* and *Fasciola hepatica*. Specific identification of the Fasciolidae from their eggs alone is hazardous.

Figure 2. The egg of *Fasciola gigantica* shown in this photomicrograph has been stained with iodine. The small operculum can easily be recognized at the upper pole of the egg (top).

Figure 3. The unstained pseudoparasite shown in this photomicrograph is *Psorospermium haeckelii*. This organism, variously known as "corpora parasitica" or "beaver body," has been found in many species of crayfish. It is occasionally found in the stools of persons who have recently ingested crayfish. It may be confused with some of the larger helminth eggs, particularly those of *Schistosoma haematobium* or *Schistosoma mansoni*, although it is readily differentiable.

Figure 4. *Psorospermium haeckelii* is shown here after staining with iodine. For over 100 years, workers have described these "spores" within the tissues of crayfish but have been unable to determine their origin and significance. This most unusual and interesting pseudoparasite must not be mistaken for a helminth egg.

(X430)

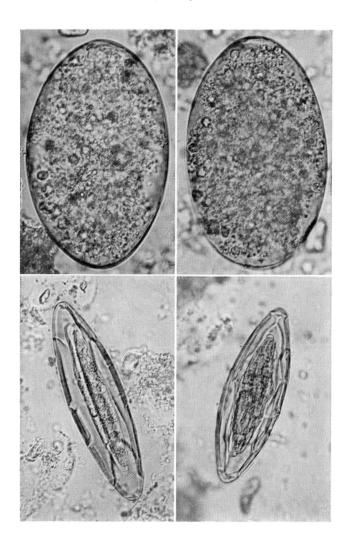

Color Plate XXXIII

Figure 1. The egg of *Capillaria philippinensis* closely resembles that of *Trichuris trichiura*. Note the pitting or striation of the outer shell, the barrel-shaped outline, and the somewhat flattened polar plugs.

Figure 2. The eggs of *Capillaria hepatica* could easily be mistaken for those of *Trichuris trichiura* or *Capillaria philippinensis*. Distinguishing features are the ovoidal configuration and the cross striations of the outer shell.

Figure 3. Photo of aspirate from an acute amebic liver abscess (symptoms less than 2 weeks). Note the dark brown color and gelatinous appearance.

Figure 4. Aspirate to show variation in appearance of an acute amebic liver abscess. Note marbled appearance.

Figure 5. Acute amebic liver abscess.

Figure 6. Acute amebic liver abscess.

Figure 7. Acute amebic liver abscess.

Figure 8. Acute amebic liver abscess.

(All Actual Size Except Top Two Which are X430)

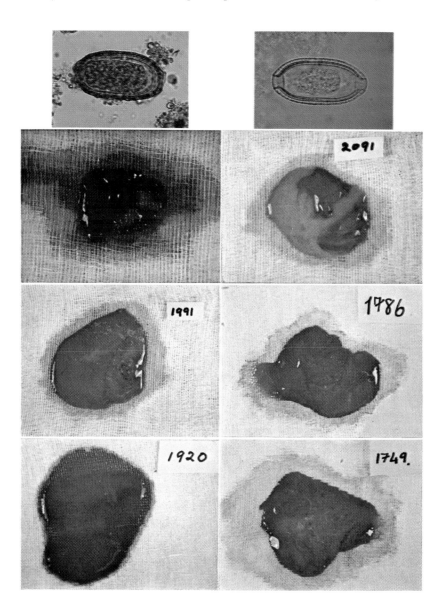

Color Plate XXXIV

Figure 1. Photo of the aspirate from subacute amebic liver abscess (symptoms for between 2 weeks and 3 months).

Figure 2. Aspirate from a subacute liver abscess.

Figure 3. Aspirate from a subacute liver abscess.

Figure 4. Aspirate from a subacute liver abscess.

Figure 5. Aspirate from a subacute liver abscess.

Figure 6. Aspirate from a chronic amebic liver abscess (symptoms for more than 3 months).

Figure 7. Aspirate from a chronic liver abscess. Note thin consistency and variable color. Compare color to Figure 8.

Figure 8. Aspirate from a chronic amebic liver abscess.

(All Actual Size)

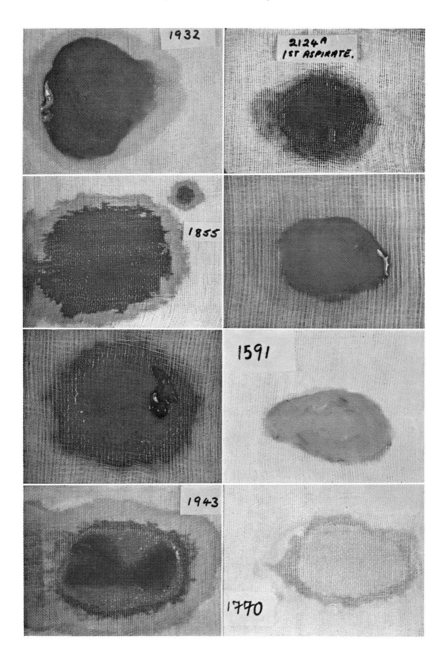

Chapter 4

THE INTESTINAL HELMINTHS

THE NEMATODES

Enterobius vermicularis

THE common pinworm is a cosmopolitan intestinal parasite, estimated to infect more than 29 million persons in North America and an additional 300 million throughout the rest of the world (updating Stoll's figures to 1974 population estimates). *E. vermicularis* is even more common in cold and temperate climates than in the tropics and is especially prevalent in groups living in crowded conditions. Pinworm infection is less common in adults than in children, in whom direct anus-to-mouth transfer of the eggs by finger contamination helps to perpetuate the infection for very long periods. This cycle of autoinfection is encouraged by the intense anal pruritus, which is foremost among the many troublesome symptoms attributed to this parasite.

The eggs are rarely passed in the feces, since the females seldom oviposit except during their nightly excursions over the anal and perianal regions. Specific diagnosis by recovery of the characteristic eggs is therefore best accomplished with the Scotch adhesive cellulose tape swab technique described on page 11. Occasionally the adult female worm will be observed crawling about the anal or perianal region and less frequently may be seen on the surface of the stool. The clinician must not rely on the observations of the individual, particularly an anxious parent, who reports seeing an adult worm in the feces. A great many such fallacious reports, which cannot be substantiated by repeated examinations, are brought to every physician. To the untrained eye, a small thread of mucus, or a vegetable fiber, attached to the surface of the stool and waving about in the water, may appear to be an actively motile "worm." Again, the moving object may be a fly maggot. It is always best to insist that such suspicious object be brought to the laboratory for accurate identification. The diagnosis of pinworm infection on the basis of such tenuous evidence is partly responsible for the exaggerated importance attached to *Enterobius* by some practitioners in this country.

The elongate, ovoidal eggs of *E. vermicularis* are flattened on one side and possess a rather thick, translucent shell. They are easily recognized and are not likely to be confused with the eggs of other species.

SEE COLOR PLATE **XXI** FOR PHOTOMICROGRAPHS DEMONSTRATING THE EGGS OF *Enterobius vermicularis.*

Ascaris lumbricoides

Of all the helminths parasitizing man, this giant intestinal roundworm is the most common and widely distributed. It is estimated from the statistics of Stoll (1947) that 4 1/2 million persons in North America are infected and that the world incidence of ascariasis to be more than one billion. *Ascaris*, largest of the common nematode parasites of man, flourishes in the warm, moist climates of temperate and tropical regions. Heavy infections of more than three fourths of the population may be found in areas where sanitation is inadequate, personal hygiene is neglected, and human feces are used as fertilizer or promiscuously deposited on the ground.

A diagnosis of *Ascaris* infection is established by recognition of the characteristic eggs in the feces, or occasionally by identification of an adult or immature roundworm that has been passed spontaneously or has been vomited. At times the adult worm is discovered on X-ray examination by the characteristic defect produced in the barium-filled intestine. The appearance is especially striking when the parasite's own intestinal tract is visualized as a thin line of ingested barium running longitudinally through the radiolucent shadow formed by its body.

Unfertilized eggs of *Ascaris* are generally larger than the fertilized eggs, and they tend to be narrower and more elongate. The external shell is very coarsely mammillated, and internally the egg is composed of a mass of highly refractile granules of variable size. The resulting appearance is quite bizarre and may cause these unfertilized eggs to be overlooked or mistaken for a plant structure.

Fertilized *Ascaris* eggs may be ovoidal or nearly spherical. The eggs are unsegmented when passed in the stool, but segmentation of the embryonic mass may begin, under favorable conditions, after standing for a short time. The thick, transparant shell of the egg has a coarse, mammillated, external albuminoid layer which is quite easily separated from the thick, smooth shell underlying it; at times this layer may never have been added. In either case, when this distinctive outer layer is absent, the egg is spoken of as being decorticated. If the appearance of such eggs is not familiar to the examiner, they may be mistaken for eggs of hookworms or *Trichostrongylus* spp. When confronted with the problem of distinguishing decorticated eggs of *Ascaris* from those of *Necator americanus* or *Trichostrongylus* spp., it is helpful to remember that the external shell of *Ascaris* is much thicker, even after the loss of the mammillated albuminoid layer. Moreover, the space between the developing embryo and the external shall is readily stained by iodine in the case of *Ascaris* but remains unstained in the other species mentioned, unless the shell has been damaged or has deteriorated.

SEE COLOR PLATES **XXI** AND **XXII** FOR PHOTOMICROGRAPHS DEMONSTRATING THE FERTILIZED AND UNFERTILIZED EGGS OF *Ascaris lumbricoides.*

Necator americanus and *Ancylostoma duodenale*

It is probable that nearly a quarter of the world's people suffer from hookwork infection, since ancient times one of the most economically disastrous diseases afflicting mankind. The human misery attributable to these parasites throughout the warm moist climates of the globe is incalcuable. *Necator americanus*, the New World hookworm, is the species prevalent in North America and large parts of South America, as well as in central and southern Africa and southern Asia. *Ancylostoma duodenale*, the Old World hookworm, predominates in the countries bordering the Mediterranean and in Japan, Korea, North China, and parts of India. Both species are found in certain other areas. No attempt should be made to distinguish the two species on the basis of the minor differences in the size of the eggs, which are otherwise morphologically identical. Since the two species may produce identical clinical manifestations, little is gained in the clinical laboratory by attempts to define exactly the geographic distribution of each.

A diagnosis of hookworm infection is established by recovery of the characteristic eggs from the stools. The ovoidal eggs have bluntly rounded ends and possess a colorless, thin hyaline shell. The shell is not stained by iodine, nor is the space between the external shell and the developing embryo, if the shell is intact and the egg has not deteriorated. The eggs are unsegmented or in an early segmentation stage when passed in the stool. However, if the specimen has been allowed to stand for a few hours in a suitably warm environment, development may have progressed to the first larval stage. In a few instances, the liberated larvae will be found and must be distinguished from those of *Strongyloides stercoralis* and the free-living *Rhabditis* spp. The long, narrow buccal chamber and the inconspicuous genital primordium characteristic of first-stage hookworm larvae contrast with the short buccal chamber and prominent genital primordium of the rhabditoid *Strongyloides* larvae. Therefore, differentation of the two species is not usually difficult.

Rhabditis hominis and related free-living rhabditoid nematode species are more difficult to distinguish from the rhabditoid hookworm larvae. *Rhabditis* spp. have a very long and more thickly cuticularized buccal chamber, and a bulbar swelling in the middle of the anterior club-shaped portion of the esophagus. These are of diagnostic value. The larvae of the free-living *Rhabditis* spp. may be considerably larger than those of either *Strongyloides* or hookworm, and larvae of *Rhabditis* spp. having greatly varying size may be present in a single stool.

SEE COLOR PLATES **XXIII** AND **XXIV** FOR PHOTOMICROGRAPHS DEMONSTRATING THE EGGS AND RHABDITOID LARVA OF *Necator americanus*, AND THE RHABDITOID LARVAE OF *Strongyloides stercoralis*, AND THE FREE-LIVING NEMATODE *Rhabditis hominis*.

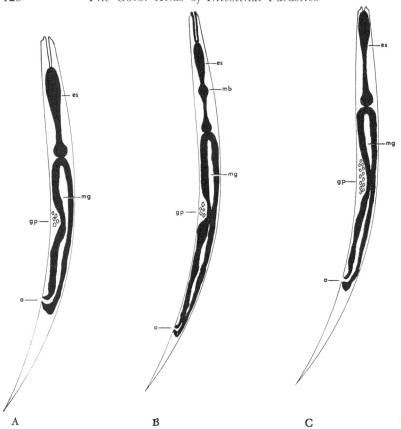

A   B   C

Diagram 6. Variations in morphology of the rhabditoid larvae of
(A) hookworm, (B) *Rhabditis* spp., and (C) *Strongyloides*. Es = esophagus;
mb = midesophageal swelling; mg = midgut; gp = germinal primordium;
a = anus.

Trichostrongylus orientalis

Reports from many parts of the world indicate that a number
of *Trichostrongylus* spp. parasitize the digestive tract of man.
Probably the most important member of the genus is *Trichostrongylus orientalis*, a common parasite in Japan, Korea,
China, and Formosa. Though a close relative of the hookworms, *Trichostrongylus* spp. infection is acquired when con-

taminated vegetables are ingested, since the larvae developing in the soil rarely, if ever, penetrate the skin. Except for a minute knob at the tip of the tail, the rhabditoid larva of *Trichostrongylus* is morphologically similar to those of hookworms, so that differentiation is often difficult.

Although the various species of *Trichostrongylus* cannot be identified from the appearance of the eggs alone, differentiation from the eggs of hookworm is not difficult. The eggs of *Trichostrongylus* resemble those of *Necator americanus*, but they are larger and more elongate, and they exhibit a characteristic tendency for one end of the egg to be somewhat pointed or elliptical rather than broadly rounded.

SEE COLOR PLATE XXIII FOR PHOTOMICROGRAPHS DEMONSTRATING THE EGGS OF *Trichostrongylus orientalis.*

Trichuris (Trichocephalus) trichiura

The whipworm, *Trichuris trichiura*, is widely distributed throughout the warm, moist climates of the world, and in tropical and subtropical areas, both the incidence and the intensity of the infection may be very high. Serious disease may result from very heavy infections, and while the patient may be relieved of a large part of the worm burden by appropriate therapy, it is very difficult to eradicate safely all the worms. As in the case of the hookworms, infection with this species may persist for several years despite the absence of reexposure.

Specific diagnosis of *Trichuris* infection is made by demonstration of the typical eggs in the patient's stool. Eggs of this helminth are characteristically barrel-shaped, with bipolar refractile intralaminar prominences, usually called polar plugs. The outer layer of the triple shell is usually bile stained. Of all the helminth eggs, this is one of the most easily recognized.

SEE COLOR PLATE XXIII FOR PHOTOMICROGRAPHS DEMONSTRATING THE EGGS OF *Trichuris trichiura.*

Capillaria philippinensis and *C. hepatica*

Intestinal capillariasis is produced by infection with the nematode *Capillaria philippinensis*, a helminth that produces eggs morphologically similar to *T. trichiura*. The infection is encountered chiefly in the coastal regions of the Philippines, where more than 1000 cases have been reported. Severe infection is accompanied by abdominal pain and diarrhea, and a fatal malabsorption state may develop.

Specific diagnosis of intestinal capillariasis is made by identification of the eggs, which have a superficial resemblance to those of *T. trichiura*. The eggs of *C. philippinensis* differ, however, in the presence of pitting, striations, and the cylindrical configuration of the outer shell. The bipolar plugs appear somewhat flattened in contrast to those of *T. trichiura*.

Capillaria hepatica is a nematode parasite chiefly of rodents although dogs, squirrels, and monkeys are occasionally infected. Rare cases of human infection have been reported, with the finding of eggs within the liver. However, eggs present in the stool are due to the consumption of infected liver in the reservoir hosts.

The eggs of *C. hepatica* resemble those of *T. trichiura* but have an outer shell that is pitted or cross striated. The egg outline is more ovoidal than that of *C. philippinensis*.

See Color Plate **XXXIII** for photomicrographs demonstrating the eggs of *Capillaria philippinensis* and *Capillaria hepatica*.

Strongyloides stercoralis

The world distribution of this important intestinal parasite is quite similar to that of hookworms. Although *Strongyloides* is generally a less common parasite, its incidence is higher than that of hookworm in some areas. Severe diarrhea may be present in some cases, and hyperinfection may produce serious disease with occasional fatalities. Autoinfection may be responsible for infections that persist for many years in the absence of any opportunity for external reinfection.

The diagnosis of intestinal strongyloidiasis is established by demonstration of the actively motile rhabditoid larvae in the feces. These larvae of *Strongyloides* may also be recovered from material obtained by duodenal drainage, when that portion of the intestinal tract is infected. Occasionally the adult parasite will be found in the stool, or in the duodenal aspirate. Very rarely will the eggs be found in the stools, since the larvae normally hatch in the tissues of the intestinal wall and work their way to the lumen, subsequently migrating down to the anus. However, when heavy infections produce mucosal ulceration and sloughing, the embryonating eggs of *Strongyloides* may occasionally appear in diarrheic stools. Under such circumstances, it may be difficult to distinguish these eggs from those of the hookworms, which are morphologically similar but somewhat larger.

The rhabditoid larvae of *Strongyloides* are readily distinguished from those of hookworms and free-living *Rhabditis* spp. by their very short buccal chamber and by the presence of a conspicuous genital primordium.

SEE COLOR PLATE XXIV FOR PHOTOMICROGRAPHS DEMONSTRATING THE EGGS AND RHABDITOID LARVA OF *Strongyloides stercoralis.*

THE CESTODES

Taenia saginata and *Taenia solium*

Infection with the beef tapeworm, *Taenia saginata,* is common in the United States, while infections with the pork tapeworm, *Taenia solium,* are rarely encountered. *Taenia saginata* has a particularly high incidence in Mohammedan countries and in Ethiopia, and is also quite prevalent in Central and South America. In most parts of the world, infections with this cosmopolitan parasite are more common than are infections with the pork tapeworm. However, the incidence of *Taenia solium* infections is high in Mexico, Central America, South America, North China, Manchuria, and India.

While important digestive symptoms, nutritional disturbances, and systemic manifestations may attend infection with *T. saginata,* very few cases of cysticercosis of man have been reported. For this reason beef tapeworm infections are much less dangerous than are those caused by *T. solium*, for the latter species frequently produces cysticercosis in man.

The eggs of *T. saginata* are morphologically indistinguishable from those of *T. solium*. Species identification must, therefore, be made by recovery of the distinctive scolex, or by study of the characteristic gravid proglottids. The eggs of *Taenia* spp. are spherical, relatively small, dark brown objects having a thick, radially striated shell. The enclosed embryo (oncosphere) possesses three pairs of hooklets, which are easily seen in fresh, ripe specimens but may be difficult to recgonize in preserved material. The thick-walled eggs are originally provided with a hyaline embryonic membrane, sometimes called a "mucous sheath." This distinctive envelope is not often present but, when seen, aids in recognition of the eggs of *Taenia* spp.

SEE COLOR PLATE **XXV** FOR PHOTOMICROGRAPHS DEMONSTRATING THE EGGS OF *Taenia* SPP.

Since the eggs of *Taneia solium* and *Taenia saginata* are not morphologically distinguishable, species differentiation is made on the basis of their scolices and proglottids (Diagram 7).

The gravid proglottids of *T. solium* are distinguished by the presence of seven to thirteen main lateral arms of the uterus on each side; those of *T. saginata* have fifteen to twenty on each side.

The scolex of *T. solium* is about 1 mm in diameter and possesses four large, deeply cupped suckers. Its prominent rostellum is armed with a double row of large and small hooklets, twenty-two to thirty-two in number. The scolex of *T. saginata* is larger, being nearly 2 mm in diameter. It also is equipped with four suckers, lacks the rostellum and rostellar hooks found in *T. solium*, and has an apical depression.

Diphyllobothrium latum

The fish tapeworm, also called the broad tapeworm, is a common parasite in many parts of the world where freshwater fish is an important item in the diet and is sometimes eaten

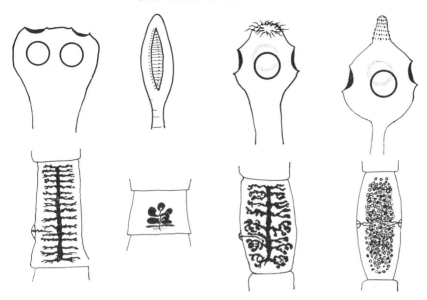

Diagram 7. The scolices (top row) and gravid proglottids of (left to right) *Taenia saginata*; *Diphyllobothrium latum*; *Taenia solium*; *Dipylidium caninum*.

raw, pickled, or insufficiently cooked. Endemic foci exist over a wide area of the subarctic and temperate zones of the northern hemisphere, including Alaska, Canada, and Scandinavian countries, the British Isles, Finland, Poland, and the U.S.S.R. Recent reports of infection arising in the Great Lakes region of the United States are lacking. *D. latum* infection is also found frequently in Switzerland, northern Italy, and parts of Central and Eastern Europe, as well as Japan, Korea, and the lake districts of Chile and Argentina. It should be remembered that infection may be acquired by eating refrigerated fish shipped from endemic areas. For this reason, infections are not uncommon in persons living hundreds of miles from any endemic foci, as in New York City.

While some persons infected with this parasite remain asymptomatic and in apparent good health, toxic manifestations or a serious anemia are not infrequently present.

The diagnosis is made by demonstration of the characteristic eggs in the feces. The eggs are operculate, ovoidal bodies having a moderately thick but rather fragile shell; they are not embryonated when passed in the feces.

The distinctive scolex of *D. latum* has a delicate, tapered oblong end and is divided by two grooves situated in the long axis. Gravid and mature progloittids have a greater width than breadth and possess a centrally placed uterus in the form of a rosette. See Diagram 7 for the mature proglotid and scolex of *D. latum*.

S<small>EE</small> C<small>OLOR</small> P<small>LATE</small> XXV <small>FOR</small> <small>PHOTOMICROGRAPHS</small> <small>DEMONSTRATING THE EGGS OF</small> *Diphyllobothrium latum.*

Hymenolepis nana

The distribution of *H. nana*, the dwarf tapeworm, is worldwide, although it is more frequently found in warm than in cold climates. In the southern United States and in Latin America, it is more common than any other tapeworm infection, and it has an especially high incidence in children. It is a common parasite in central and southern Europe, the U.S.S.R., and India. A very large number of worms may be present, often as a result of internal autoinfection, and in such cases, pronounced intestinal disturbances as well as toxic symptoms may appear.

Diagnosis is based on recognition of the characteristic eggs passed in the feces. The eggs are spherical, or nearly spherical, hyaline bodies having a smooth, thin outer shell. The six-hooked oncosphere is contained in a tough inner envelope marked by two polar thickenings, from each of which arise four to eight threadlike polar filaments.

S<small>EE</small> C<small>OLOR</small> P<small>LATE</small> XXV <small>FOR</small> <small>PHOTOMICROGRAPHS</small> <small>DEMONSTRATING THE EGGS OF</small> *Hymenolepis nana.*

Hymenolepis diminuta

Infections with the rat tapeworm, *H. diminuta*, are not frequently encountered in man. However, cases have been reported from many parts of the world, including more than a dozen of the states in the U.S.A. The largest number of authentic human cases have been reported from India, the

U.S.S.R., Japan, Italy, and the southern United States. Most patients harboring this parasite experience few if any symptoms, though cachexia may be present if the infection is heavy. The diagnosis of *H. diminuta* infection is established by recovery of the typical eggs from the stool. They are considerably larger than those of *H. nana* and lack the polar filaments found in that species. Eggs of *H. diminuta* are spherical or slightly ovoidal in shape, and yellowish brown in color. The inner membrane surrounding the six-hooked oncosphere is separated from the transparent outer shell by a rather wide space filled with a colorless, gelantinous matrix.

SEE COLOR PLATE XXV FOR PHOTOMICROGRAPHS DEMONSTRATING THE EGGS OF *Hymenolepis diminuta.*

Dipylidium caninum

Dipylidium caninum has a worldwide distribution and is a common organism parasitizing cats and dogs. Man, and particularly children, become infected through the accidental ingestion of fleas containing cysticercoid larvae. The egg packets of *D. caninum* are seldom seen and have little diagnostic value. The mature proglottid, passed singly or in chains in the stool, is longer than it is wide. Containing two sets of male and female reproductive organs and two uterine pores, the proglottids are characteristic and should offer no difficulties in diagnosis. The scolex is cone shaped and contains four suckers and a rostellum with six small circles of hooklets. See Diagram 7 for the mature proglottid and scolex of *D. caninum.*

THE TREMATODES

Clonorchis (Opisthorchis) sinensis

The Chinese liver fluke, *C. sinenis*, is endemic in Japan, Korea, China, Taiwan, and Vietnam. It is now estimated from Stoll's figures that more than 30 million persons living in eastern Asia are infected with this parasite. It is occasionally found in Orientals living in the western hemisphere, and in persons who have traveled or resided for a time in one of the endemic areas.

Persons lightly infected with *C. sinensis* are usually asymptomatic. The severity of the symptoms depends upon the number of worms present and the duration of the infection, which may exceed a period of twenty years. Heavy infections often result from repeated or continuous exposure over a period of many years. In these cases, epithelial hyperplasia, inflammatory changes, and fibrosis in the biliary duct system lead to progressive impairment of hepatic function and culminate in portal cirrhosis, which may prove fatal.

A diagnosis of clonorchiasis is established by demonstration of the characteristic eggs in the feces, or in material obtained by duodenal aspiration. The eggs of *C. sinensis* closely resemble those of the heterophyids, *Heterophyes heterophyes* and *Metagonimus yokogawai*. The tiny eggs are characteristically ovoidal or pyriform in shape and have a rather thick, hard shell. The prominent, distinctly convex operculum fits snugly into a flared portion of the shell that produces the conspicuous shoulders that are a unique and characteristic feature of the eggs of this species. A short, comma-shaped process is frequently present at the abopercular end of the egg. When seen, this knob, or boss, is a helpful and distinctive morphologic feature. *Clonorchis sinensis* and certain other trematodes not infrequently produce anomalous or incomplete eggs. Such abnormal eggs of *Clonorchis* may lack the morphologic characteristics that usually serve to distinguish them from the eggs of *Metagonimus yokogawai* and certain other trematodes.

SEE COLOR PLATES **XXVII** FOR PHOTOMICROGRAPHS DEMONSTRATING THE EGGS OF *Clonorchis sinensis.*

Heterophyes heterophyes and *Metagonimus yokogawai*

The heterophyids, *Heterophyes heterophyes* and *Metagonimus yokogawai*, are tiny intestinal flukes found frequently in the Far East. *Heterophyes* is common in the Nile Delta, and several endemic foci are present in Japan, Korea, China, Taiwan, and the Philippines. *Metagonimus* is the most prevalent heterophyid in Japan, Korea, and the Maritime Provinces of the U.S.S.R., Siberia, and the Balkan States. *Metagonimus* has also been reported in Spain, and both species have been found in Israel.

Many persons infected with these flukes are asymptomatic, but at times, particularly when the infection is heavy, diarrhea and abdominal discomfort may be present. Symptoms are probably the result of mucosal inflammatory reaction at the sites of attachment of the worms in the intestine.

The diagnosis of infection due to these two species is made by recognition of the eggs in the patient's stools. The tiny heterophyid eggs are differentiated with great difficulty from each other and from those of *Clonorchis sinensis*. In general, the heterophyid eggs are slightly smaller than those of *C. sinensis* and lack the prominent flare ("shouldering") at the line of cleavage between the shell and the operculum. The operculum is much less conspicuous in the eggs of *Heterophyes* and *Metagnonimus* than in those of *C. sinensis*, and a definite knob, or boss, at the abopercular end of the shell is often lacking.

SEE COLOR PLATE **XXVII** FOR PHOTOMICROGRAPHS DEMONSTRATING THE EGGS OF *Heterophyes heterophyes* AND *Metagonimus yokogawai.*

Echinostomatoidea and *Paramphistomatoidea*

A number of digenetic trematodes belonging to the superfamily Echinostomatoidea parasitize man in the Philippines, Japan, Taiwan, and certain other areas in Asia and the Far East. The most important species is *Echinostoma ilocanum*, a common intestinal fluke in parts of the Philippines and Celebes. A related species, *Echinochasmus perfoliatus*, is a common intestinal parasite of dogs and cats in parts of central Europe, Asia, and the Far East. Infection in man has been reported from Japan.

The diagnosis of echinostome infection is made by recovery of the eggs from the stool. These eggs are generally ovoidal or ellipsoidal and operculate, and are immature when passed. However, the eggs of the echinostomes have little specific diagnostic value, being difficult to distinguish from each other and from the larger ones of *Fasciola hepatica* and *Fasciolopsis buski*. Identification is best made from study of the adult forms. A photomicrograph of an echinostome egg, believed to be that of *Echinochasmus perfoliatus*, is shown in Figure 1 of Color Plate XXVIII.

Gastrodiscoides hominis, a digenetic trematode of the superfamily Paramphistomatoidea, is a common intestinal fluke in parts of India, Assam, and Vietnam. Infection with this species produces a mucous diarrhea. A photomicrograph of a paramphistomid egg, believed to be that of *Gastrodiscoides hominis*, is shown in Figure 2 of Color Plate XXVIII.

Paragonimus westermani and *Paragonimus kellicotti*

The Oriental lung fluke, *P. westermani*, is common in many parts of the Far East. Heavily infected populations occur in Japan, Korea, Taiwan, China, Formosa, Thailand, Malaya, and in many of the islands of the South and Southwest Pacific. Cases have also been reported from parts of Africa and South America, including Peru, Colombia, and Ecuador.

This important parasite produces serious pulmonary disease with occasional fatalities. There are also, in many instances, lesions produced by the presence of the worms in the abdominal viscera, brain, and subcutaneous tissues. The characteristic eggs, upon which specific diagnosis is based, may be recovered from the sputum. They are also frequently present in the feces, having been swallowed with the sputum. At times the worms lodge in the intestinal wall and evoke diarrhea, accompanied by the passage of many eggs in the stools.

The eggs are broadly ovoidal in shape, with the maximum width nearer the operculum than the equator of the egg. There is a characteristic thickening of the shell at the abopercular end of the egg. The easily recognizable operculum is somewhat flattened.

While *P. westermani* is the species responsible for virtually all human cases of paragonimiasis, it is interesting that the single human infection recorded from North America was caused by *P. kellicotti*, a closely related lung fluke. This species is commonly found in mink and has been reported in a number of other wild and domestic animals in more than a dozen states of the U.S.A. and in Canada. The eggs of this species are morphologically similar to those of *P. westermani* but are more regularly ovoidal and lack the marked degree of thickening of the shell at the aborpercular end of the egg.

SEE COLOR PLATE **XXVIII** FOR PHOTOMICROGRAPHS DEMONSTRATING THE EGGS OF *Paragonimus westermani* AND *Paragonimus kellicotti.*

Dicrocoelium dendriticum

The lancet fluke, *D. dendriticum*, is a common parasite in the biliary passages of sheep and other herbivorous and omnivorous mammals in many parts of the world. A relatively few authentic cases of human infection have been reported from parts of Europe, North Africa, and the Far East. In many instances the eggs of this fluke are found in the feces as a result of the ingestion of infected sheep or goat livers, and no true infection exists. Spurious infections can be excluded by repeated examinations of the feces while the patient's diet is controlled. It is understandable that genuine human cases of dicroceliasis are rare, since the peculiar life cycle of this species requires that man must accidentally ingest an infected ant in order to acquire the infection! Persons infected with this parasite may experience a variety of digestive and systemic symptoms, and liver enlargement may occur.

The diagnosis of *D. dendriticum* infection is established by demonstration of the characteristic eggs in the patient's stool, but only if adequate precautions have been taken to exclude spurious infection. The rather small eggs of this species are ovoidal, thick shelled, operculate, and a deep golden brown in color.

SEE COLOR PLATE **XXVIII** FOR A PHOTOMICROGRAPH DEMONSTRATING THE EGG OF *Dicrocoelium dendriticum.*

Macracanthorhynchus hirudinaceus

This unique species, a member of the phylum Acanthocephala, is admittedly out of place among the trematodes, but it is placed here for technical reasons which prevented its being located elsewhere in the photographic series.

M. hirudinaceus is a cosmopolitan intestinal parasite in pigs. Human infection has been reported once, and in a few instances the eggs have been recovered from human stools. It is probable that in most, if not all, of these cases the infection was spurious. In order to acquire the infection, man must actually ingest the arthropod intermediate host, one of several species of beetles. Clinical data on human infection are very meager.

Photomicrographs of the eggs of *M. hirudinaceus* are shown in Figures 7 and 8 of Color Plate XXVIII.

Schistosoma mansoni

Manson's blood fluke is an exceedingly common and important trematode species, estimated from Stoll's figures (1947) to parasitize nearly 48 million persons throughout Africa and tropical America. *S. mansoni* is widely distributed over large areas in central Africa and is also found in Madagascar and Arabia. It is highly prevalent in central and northeastern Brazil, and important edemic foci exist in Venezuela, Surinam, the Dominican Republic, and other parts of the West Indies. Of particular interest is the presence of numerous endemic areas in Puerto Rico, where the incidence of the disease is very high. In recent years there has been a heavy influx of infected Puerto Ricans into New York and Chicago, and to a lesser degree into certain other large cities of the United States. As a result, schistosomiasis mansoni has become an important clinical problem in those areas. Fortunately, evidence presently available indicates a lack of propagation of the infection in North America.

The protean clinical manifestations of Manson's intestinal schistosomiasis vary with the number of parasites involved, the stage of the disease, and constitutional factors that determine the response of the individual host. The colon and rectum are the organs primarily involved in *S. mansoni* infections, but fibrotic reactions around the eggs accumulated in the periportal tissues of the liver are responsible for the gradual development of full-blown portal cirrhosis. This is the most serious end result of the disease in its chronic stage, and the prognosis in such cases is very poor.

This laboratory diagnosis of *S. mansoni* infection becomes possible as soon as egg extrusion has begun, usually some seven or more weeks after exposure. The large, elongate, ovoidal eggs possessing a prominent lateral spine are among the most easily recognized of all the helminth eggs. They are passed in moderately large numbers during the acute stages of the disease, particularly when the typical schistomsomal dysentery is present. As this stage the eggs are easily demonstrable in the stools without use of concentration techniques. During the chronic stage of the disease, the fibrosis of the intestinal wall may prevent all but a few eggs from appearing in the feces. In these cases the use of the formalin-ether concentration technique may be very helpful. The eggs will not be recovered by the zinc suflate concentration method, since they do not float and are often ruptured. In chronic cases where eggs cannot be found in the feces, the rectal biopsy may be valuable. Fresh tissue is teased apart, floated in normal saline, flattened, and promptly examined under the microscope. The distinctive eggs are frequently present in considerable numbers, even when a rectal lesion is not visible and the biopsy is made blindly.

See Color Plates **XXIX** and **XXX** for photomicrographs demonstrating the eggs of *Schistosoma mansoni.*

Schistonsoma haematobium

This species, causing urinary schistosomiasis, shows a pronounced tendency to occupy the venous plexuses of the urinary bladder and adjacent pelvic organs. For the most part the disease is confined to Africa and its environs, with extensive endemic foci throughout the continent. The entire valley of the Nile is a hyperendemic area. Endemic foci exist also in Madagascar, southern Portugal, Cyprus, and Asia Minor. It is estimated from Stoll's figures that nearly 64 million persons are infected with *S. haematobium*.

The clincial manifestations of schistosomiasis haematobia differ from those due to *S. mansoni* or *S. japonicum* only in that involvement is predominately in the bladder and adjacent organs, so that symptoms are related chiefly to the genitourinary tract. Hepatic involvement is rare in *S. haematobium* infections, but it is common for eggs to be carried to the lungs, where they are filtered out and produce pulmonary fibrosis. Rectal involvement is also relatively common in Africa.

A specific diagnosis of *S. haematobium* infection is established by demonstration of the characteristic terminal-spined eggs in the urine or the stool, or in biopsy material from the vesical or rectal mucosa. Sedimentation or centrifugation of the urine is usually necessary to recover the eggs, and they are especially likely to be found if the blood and pus discharged at the end of micturition are examined. Eggs are present less frequently, and often in smaller numbers, in the stools. However, they may be found if the formalin-ether concentration technique is used. Eggs are perhaps more frequently found in biopsy snippings from the bladder or rectal mucosa in chronic infections.

SEE COLOR PLATE **XXIX** FOR PHOTOMICROGRAPHS DEMONSTRATING THE EGGS OF *Schistosoma haematobium.*

Schistosoma japonicum

Infections caused by the Oriental blood fluke, *S. japonicum*, are limited to the Far East. The most heavily endemic areas are found in China, where infection is especially prevalent along the basin of the Yangtze river, and in the Philippines. Important endemic foci also exist in other parts of China, in Japan, and in one area in the Celebes. Extrapolating from Stoll's figures, it is estimated that the total incidence of schistosomiasis japonica approaches 73 million persons.

The adult worms of this species inhabit the branches of the superior mesenteric vein, and the exceptionally large numbers of eggs are deposited in the venules of the intestinal mucosa and submucosa. The eggs readily traverse the bowel wall to the intestinal lumen and are dischared in the feces. Extensive tissue damage is produced in the intestinal tract and in the liver, and less frequently in the spleen, lungs, and brain. The clinical manifestations are appropriately diverse and may be very severe. The prognosis in this parasitic infection is poor, unless adequate and specific treatment is administered early in the course of the disease, prior to the development of irreparable damage to the liver and other vital organs.

The specific diagnosis of *S. japonicum* infection is dependent upon recovery of the characteristic eggs in the stools, or their demonstration in the tissue obtained by biopsy of the rectal mucosa. The formalin-ether concentration technique for recovery of the eggs from the feces is of considerable value, especially in the chronic cases and in lightly infected persons. The zinc sulfate technique fails to recover most of the eggs of this species and should not be used when *S. japonicum* is suspected.

The eggs of *S. japonicum* are regularly ovoidal in shape and are smaller and proportionately broader than those of the other two schistosomes. They are usually described as having an abbreviated lateral spine, which may appear as a tiny recurved hook, visible only when the egg is properly oriented and is viewed in a suitable projection. It is therefore rarely seen and should not be considered a *sine qua non* in identifying eggs of this species. Blood cells, tissue cells, and similar debris are frequently seen adhering to the shell of the eggs of *S. japonicum*.

SEE COLOR PLATE XXX FOR PHOTOMICROGRAPHS DEMONSTRATING THE EGGS OF *Schistosoma japonicum.*

Fasciolopsis buski

The giant intestinal fluke, *F. buski*, is estimated to infect 16 million persons in eastern Asia and the southwest Pacific. It is common throughout central and southern China, Taiwan, and Thailand, and in parts of Indonesia and India.

Pronounced inflammation and deep ulceration of the intestinal mucosa may develop at the site of attachment of the large, fleshy worms. In heavy infections, intestinal obstruction may occur in addition to the profound intoxication caused by absorption of the worm's metabolites. While the prognosis is fairly good in light infections and early cases that are properly treated, symptoms are very severe in late cases with heavy infections, and death is not uncommon.

A specific diagnosis of fasciolopsiasis is made by recognition of the large, ovoidal, operculate eggs, which are passed in great numbers of feces. Although the eggs of the species are generally a little larger than those of *Fasciola hepatica,* there is considerable overlapping, and no reliable morphologic differences exist to permit positive species identification. Specific differentiation of the Fasciolidae from their eggs alone is not possible in individual cases, despite minor differences that can be detected when studying photomicrographs of the three species placed side by side.

SEE COLOR PLATES XXX AND XXXI FOR PHOTOMICROGRAPHS DEMONSTRATING THE EGGS OF *Fasciolopsis buski.*

Fasciola hepatica

The sheep liver fluke, *Fasciola hepatica,* is prevalent in the herbivorous mammals of sheep-raising countries throughout the world. Human infections have been reported from many parts of South America, Europe, China, the U.S.S.R., Africa, and Latin America. The incidence of human infection with this parasite is growing in frequency and importance in Cuba and the Caribbean area, as well as in several Mediteranean countries. Many enzotic foci exist in the southern, western, and northern portions of the United States. The authors have encountered one case of fascioliasis hepatica, the diagnosis having been established by identification of an adult fluke removed from the common bile duct at the time of cholecystectomy, performed for chronic cholecystitis and cholelithiasis. The infection was apparently incurred in California. To our knowledge, this is the first proven human infection with this parasite recorded in this country.

The presence of numbers of flukes in the biliary duct system may result in extensive and serious damage to the liver parenchyma as well as to the biliary tree. In heavy infections, or when the liver has been seriously damaged before chemotherapy has been instituted, the prognosis is grave.

The diagnosis of *F. hepatica* infection is based upon recovery of the characteristic eggs from the patient's stool. The large, ovoidal, operculate eggs cannot be differentiated with certainty from the morphologically similar eggs of certain echinostomes, or from those of the other Fasciolidae.

SEE COLOR PLATE **XXXI** FOR PHOTOMICROGRAPHS DEMONSTRATING THE EGGS OF *Fasicola hepatica.*

Fasciola gigantica

The giant liver fluke, *F. gigantica*, is a common parasite of cattle and other herbivorous mammals in Asia, Africa, and Hawaii. Human infections with this species have been reported from West Africa, Indochina, the U.S.S.R., and Hawaii.

The clinical manifestations and pathologic aspects of infection with this parasite are similar to those seen in *Fasciola hepatica* infections. The diagnosis of *F. gigantica* infection is made upon recovery of the huge, operculate eggs from the feces. The eggs of *F. gigantica* are the largest of the helminth eggs but are not otherwise distinguishable from those of *F. hepatica.*

SEE COLOR PLATE **XXXII** FOR PHOTOMICROGRAPHS DEMONSTRATING THE EGGS OF *Fasciola gigantica.*

Chapter 5

CONFUSING OBJECTS FOUND IN FECES

THE most common mistake of the inadequately trained technician is the erroneous identification of some object in the stool as an intestinal parasite. To avoid these errors, it is of paramount importance that the technician be imbued with the idea that *rigid morphologic criteria must govern identification of an organism.* When he finds objects that are apparently parasitic structures but which do not conform exactly with the authoritative descriptions, diagrams, or photomicrographs, the chances are that he is mistaken.

An all-inclusive term for these confusing objects has not yet been devised. The word "artifact" has been applied to the entire group but, in the strictest sense, should be used to designate artificial modifications of the stool such as the presence of mineral oil droplets. The term "spurious parasite" has been used to designate free-living animals, occasionally parasitic to other hosts, which transit the human intestinal tract and are found by accident on stool examination. Further, the term "commensal" is reserved for those organisms which benefit from their inhabitation of the intestinal tract but which neither harm nor benefit their host. It is probably better that one should try to name or categorize the confusing objects found on stool examination and leave to the specialist in semantics the invention of more appropriate terminology.

Objects Mistaken for Protozoa

Surprisingly enough, the *polymorphonuclear leucocyte* is probably the most commonly misinterpreted structure found in the feces. This ubiquitous cell can readily masquerade as a protozoan cyst or trophozoite. In permanently stained slides the nuclei are seen frequently as rounded bodies with peripheral chromatin and a central mass of deeply-staining material. The appearance of four such nuclei, all with apparent "karyosomes," often triggers a chain of events that begins with the deceived technician and ends with certain cases of "incurable" amebiasis which dot the medical literature. The student and technician alike should examine carefully the nuclear-cytoplasmic ratio in suspect cases. The presence of relatively large nuclei in relation to the total structure (see Color Plate I, Fig. 1, and Color Plate XIX, Fig. 5, for examples) should immediately suggest the presence of a polymorphonuclear leucocyte. The absence of a regular, rounded cyst wall with a surrounding clear zone, chromatoidal material, and the characteristic cytoplasm of an amebic cyst should confirm the suspicion.

Phagocytes, often found in mucopurulent stool specimens, may be confused with a trophozoite of *Entamoeba histolytica*, as these macrophages may ingest red blood cells and exhibit sluggish motility (see Color Plates, I, XVIII, and XIX for examples). In permanently stained preparations, the typical nucleus of *Entamoeba* spp. is the single most important criterion that should be sought. In wet mounts, the large size of the phagocyte, its granular, debris-filled cytoplasm and sluggish motility are additional features that serve to distinguish it from a pathogenic amebic trophozoite.

Blastocystis hominis is a structure commonly found in stool specimens, and it can confuse the inexperienced examiner. It was once believed to be a yeast; recent studies indicate that it may be a protozoan. Nevertheless, *B. hominis* has not been incriminated in any disease process. This organism has a highly refractile and apparently double-contoured wall. It contains a large central structureless mass, which is surrounded by a number of refractile bodies that are interspersed between the mass and the outer wall. In permanent smears these bodies stain quite deeply. Figures 1, 2, and 3 of Color Plate XIX demonstrate the morphology and marked variation in size of *Blastocystis hominis*. Without attention to morphologic details, this yeast could be confused with an immature amebic cyst.

Oil or fat droplets are highly refractile and will sometimes be mistaken for an amebic cyst if a search for internal structure is not undertaken. *Yeasts* may mimic amebic cysts, particularly those of *Endolimax nana*, but can be differentiated easily by their lack of characteristic nuclei in stained preparations. *Starch granules* may be recognized by their irregular shape, the presence of surface markings, and the staining reaction with iodine. The spores of certain *fungi* such as corn smut (see Color Plate XXVII, Fig. 2) are occasionally seen but lack the internal morphologic features that could be confused with protozoan forms.

Coprozoic protozoans may rarely be encountered in contaminated or improperly preserved stool specimens. Of these, the *free-living amebae* should be identified in their cystic forms by their unusually thick cyst wall, and in the trophozoite stage by their large size and the presence of one or more contractile vacuoles. *Coprozoic Ciliata* usually belonging to the genera *Chilodon* or *Cyclidium* can be confused with *Balantidium coli*. The free-living and coprozoic ciliates are generally much smaller than *B. coli* and are not apt to possess a large macronucleus having the distinctive shape of that seen in the pathogenic species. To eliminate such confusing organisms, water that has been exposed to air should not be mixed with feces, as a contamination with such coprozoic protozoans is apt to occur.

A wide variety of unclassified *plant material* can frequently cause the novice to speculate but will seldom give rise to serious question if the diagnostic morphologic features of the various intestinal parasites are sought. An example of such a plant form is seen in Figure 8 of Color Plate XVIII. The plant structure in Color Plate XX, Figure 3, probably is a *pollen grain*. *Diatoms*, a fresh and salt water algae with a silicaceous outer wall, are common constitutents of the various commercial scouring powders and hence find their way into the digestive tract. Color Plate XXVII, Figure 1, and Color Plate XVIII, Figure 7, probably are diatoms demonstrating geometric and highly refractile surface markings.

Objects Mistaken for Helminths

Scarcely a week goes by when a technician is not called upon to identify certain "wormlike objects" in a stool sample.

Mucous shreds or casts and *vegetable* fibers are frequently submitted by a frightened patient who visualizes some dangerous parasite in the stringlike material. Gross inspection will, of course, easily verify the lack of segmentation or uterine or internal structure characteristic of the various helminths. Reassurance of the patient may be more difficult.

Microscopic plant structures also often confuse the novice technician but should cause no real difficulty. Color Plate XXVI, Figures 1 and 8, demonstrate the typical structure of plant cells, while Figures 3 and 4 show the typical morphology of a *stone cell.* Found in a wide variety of plants, *stone cells* have a thickened hyaline wall and irregular shape. They contribute to the gritty texture of pears and comprise nearly the entirety of nutshells. In some plants species the *stone cells* have radial striations, which are seen in the outer wall — a finding that might cause confusion because of the superifical resemblance to the eggs of *Taenia* spp. A spiral vessel, or "vegetable spiral," a component of plant xylem, is shown in Color Plate XXVI, Figure 2. Such structures are formed from a series of lignified cylindrical cells. Color Plate XXVI, Figure 5, shows a *plant hair* which on casual inspection might be mistaken for a rhabditiform larva of *Strongyloides stercoralis.* However, the minute central canal that runs the entire length of the structure, and its tapered shape, should serve as important differential landmarks.

Even more difficult to differentiate from the rhabditiform larvae of *Strongyloides* are the free-living *Rhabditis* spp. (see Color Plate XXIV, Figs, 7 and 8). These occasional stool contaminants are differentiated from the rhabditiform larvae of hookworm and *Strongyloides* by their great variation in size, long and thickly cuticularized buccal chamber, and the configuration of the esophagus (see Diagram 6).

Spurious parasites are probably the most difficult to detect but should be considered whenever the technician encounters any form that is not commonly a parasite of man. As in the case of the lancet fluke, *Dicrocoelium dendriticum,* where eggs in the feces are found as a result of ingestion of infected liver, spurious parasitism can be excluded by repeated examination of the feces while the diet is controlled. Certainly, before a "new" parasite is suspected, such a test should be performed. *Psorospermium haeckelii*, an unclassified object found in the muscle of crayfish (see Color Plate XXXII, Figs. 3 and 4), can probably be classed as a pseudoparasite because of its suspiciously organic structure. This form is occasionally found in the stool after a patient has ingested crayfish and could cause confusion with some of the larger helminth eggs — notably that of *Schistosoma haematobium*.

REFERENCES

Albach, R.A., and Booden, T.: Amoebae. In Krier, J. (Ed.): *Parasitic Protozoa*, Volume II. New York, Acad Pr, 1978, pp. 455-506.

Alicna, A.D., and Fadell, B.J.: The advantage of purgation in recovery of intestinal parasites of their eggs. *Am J Clin Pathol, 31:*139-141, 1959.

Binford, C.H., and Connor, C.H.: *Pathology of Tropical and Extraordinary Diseases*, Volumes I and II. Washington, D.C., Armed Forces Institute of Pathology, 1976.

Boeck, W.C., and Drbohlav, J.: The cultivation of endamoeba histolytica. *Am J Hyg, 5:*371-407, 1925

Boonpucknavig, S., and Navin, R.C.: Serological diagnosis of amebiasis by immunofluorescence. *J Clin Pathol, 20:*875-878, 1967.

Brooke, M.M.: *Amebiasis, Methods in Laboratory Diagnosis*. Public Health Service Manual, 1958.

Brook, M.M., and Goldman, M.: Polyvinyl alcohol-fixative as a preservative and adhesive for protozoa in dysenteric stools and other liquid materials. *J Lab Clin Med, 34(11):*1554-1560, 1949.

Cleveland, L.R., and Collier, J.: Various improvements in the cultivation of endamoeba histolytica. *Am J Hyg, 12:*606-613, 1930.

Diamond, L.S.: Axenic cultivation of Entamoeba histolytica. *Science, 134:*336-337, 1961.

Diamond, L.S., Harlow, D.R., and Cunnick, C.C.: A new medium for the axenic cultivation of *Entamoeba histolytica* and other *Entamoeba. Trans R Soc Trop Med Hyg. 72(4):*431-432, 1978.

Dobell, C., and O'Connors, F.W.: *The Intestinal Protozoa of Man*. London, John Bale and Sons, 1921.

Editorial. Intestinal capillariasis. A new disease of man. *Lancet, 1:*587-588, 1973.

Elsdon-Dew, R.: The pathogenicity of Entamoeba histolytica. *South Afr Med J, 27:*504-506, 1953.

Faust, E.C., D'Antoni, J.S., Odom, V., Miller, M.J., Peres, C., Sawitz, W.G., Thomen, L., Tobie, J., and Walker, J.H.: A critical study of clinical laboratory technics for the diagnosis of protozoan cysts and helminth eggs in feces. *Am J Trop Med, 18:*169-183, 1938.

Faust, E.C., Russell, F.P., and Jung, C.R.: *Craig and Faust's Clinical Parasitology*, 8th ed. Philadelphia, Lea & Febiger, 1970.

Fresh, J.W., Cross, J.H., Reyes, V., et al.: Necropsy findings in intestinal capillariasis. *Am J Trop Med, 21:*169-173, 1972.

Goldman, M.: Microfluorimetric evidence of antigenic difference between

Entamoeba histolytica and Entamoeba hartmanni. *Proc Soc Exp Biol Med, 102:*189-191, 1959.

Goldman, M.: *Entamoeba histolytica*-like amoebae occurring in man. *Bull WHO, 40:*355-364, 1969.

Gomori, G.: A rapid one-step trichrome stain. *Am J Clin Pathol, 20:*661-664, 1950.

Hartmann, D.P., Ghadirian, E., and Meerovitch, E.: Enzyme-linked Immunosorbant Assay (ELISA) and Indirect Hemagglutination (IHA) test in the serodiagnosis of experimental hepatic amebiasis. *J Parasitol, 66(2):*344-345, 1980.

Holman, R.M., and Robbins, W.W.: *The Textbook of General Botany.* New York, Wiley, 1938.

Kagan, I.G., and Norman, L.: Serodiagnosis of parasitic diseases. In Blair, J.E., Lennette, E.H., and Truant, J.P. (Eds.): *Manual of Clinical Microbiology.* Baltimore, Williams, & Wilkins, 1970, pp. 453-486.

Kean, B.H. and Malloch, C.L.: The neglected ameba: *Dietamoeba fragilis.* A report of 100 "pure" infections. *Am J Dig Dis, 2(9):*735-746, 1966.

Kessel, J.F., and Johnstone, H.G.: The occurrence of Entamoeba polecki, Prowazek 1912, in Macaca mulatta and man. *Am J Trop Med, 29:*311-317, 1949.

Kessel, J.F., Lewis, W.P., Pasquel, C.H., and Turner, J.A.: Indirect hemagglutination and complement fixation tests in amebiasis. *Am J Trop Med Hyg, 14:*540-550, 1965.

Kessel, J.F., Lewis, W.P., Solomon, M., and Kim, H.: Preliminary report on hemagglutination test for Entamoebae. *Proc Soc Exp Biol Med, 106:*2:409-413, 1961.

Krupp, I.M.: A comparison of counter-immunoelectrophoresis with other serologic tests in the diagnosis of amebiasis. *Am J Trop Med, 23:*27-30, 1974.

Kulda, J., and Nohynkova, E.: *Giardia* and giardiasis. In Krier, J. (Ed.): *Parasitic Protozoa,* Volume II. New York, Acad Pr, 1978.

Marcial-Rojas, R.A.: *Pathology of Protozoal and Helminthic Diseases.* Baltimore, Williams & Wilkins, 1971.

Miller, L.H., and Brown, H.W.: The serologic diagnosis of parasitic infections in medical practice. *Ann Intern Med, 71:* 983-992, 1969.

Morris, M.N., Powell, S.J., and Eldson-Dew, R.: Latex agglutination test for invasive amoebiasis. *Lancet, 1:*1362-1363, 1970.

Norman, L., and Brooke, M.M.: The effectiveness of the PVA-fixative technique in revealing intestinal amebae in diagnostic cultures. *Am J Trop Med Hyg, 4(3):*479-482, 1955.

Powell, S.J., Maddison, S.E., Wilmot, A.J., et al.: Amoebic gel-diffusion precipitin test. Clinical evaluation in amoebic liver disease. *Lancet, 2:*602-603, 1965.

Ritchie, L.S.: An ether sedimentation technique for routine stool examinations. *Bull US Army Med Dept, 8:*326, 1948.

Sawitz, W.G., and Faust, E.C.: The probability of detecting intestinal protozoa by successive stool examinations. *Am J Trop Med, 22:* 131-136, 1942.

Sapero, J.J., and Lawless, D.K.: The MIF stain preservation technic for the identification of intestinal protozoa. *Am J Trop Med Hyg,* 2:613-619, 1953.

Stoll, N.R.: This wormy world. *J Parasital, 33:*1-18, 1947.

Visvesvana, C.S., Smith, P.D., Healy, G.R., and Brown, W.R.: An immunofluorescence test to detect serum antibodies to *Giardia lambila. Ann Int Med, 93:*802-805, 1980.

Wenyon, C.M.: *Protozoology.* London, Baillere, Tindall, and Cox, 1926.

Wheatley, W.B.: Rapid stain for intestinal amebae and flagellates. *Am J Clin Pathol 21:*990-993, 1951.

Zierdt, C.H.: *Blastocystis hominis,* an intestinal protozoan parasite of man. *Public Health Lab, 36:*147-160, 1978.

INDEX